Forensic Nursing and Mental Disorder in Clinical Practice

To the memory of Tony Hillis

Commissioning editor: Mary Seager
Desk editor: Deena Burgess
Production controller: Anthony Read
Development editor: Caroline Savage
Cover designer: Helen Brockway

Forensic Nursing and Mental Disorder in Clinical Practice

Edited by

Norman McClelland, Martin Humphreys, Lorraine Conlon, Tony Hillis

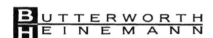

OXFORD   AUCKLAND   BOSTON   JOHANNESBURG   MELBOURNE   NEW DELHI

Butterworth-Heinemann
Linacre House, Jordan Hill, Oxford OX2 8DP
225 Wildwood Avenue, Woburn, MA 01801-2041
A division of Reed Educational and Professional Publishing Ltd

$\mathcal{R}$ A member of the Reed Elsevier plc group

First published 2001

© Reed Educational and Professional Publishing Ltd 2001

British Library Cataloguing in Publication Data
Forensic nursing and mental disorder in clinical practice
   1.   Forensic psychiatric nursing
   I.   McClelland, Norman
   610.7'368

ISBN 0 7506 4309 9

Library of Congress Cataloguing in Publication Data
Forensic nursing and mental disorder in clinical practice/edited by Norman
   McClelland ... [et al.].
   p.; cm.
   Includes bibliographical references and index.
   ISBN 0 7506 4309 9
   1.   Forensic psychiatric nursing. I.   McClelland, Norman.
   [DNLM: 1.   Mental Disorders – nursing.   2.   Forensic Psychiatry. WY
   160F7152]
   RA1155.F67
   614'.1–dc21   00–054371

Transferred to digital printing 2006

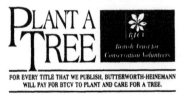

Contents

Contributors vii

Acknowledgements ix

Foreword xi
by Rosemarie V. Cope

Introduction xiii
Gina Hillis

1 Referral to admission 1
   Phil Walsh, Alex Kearns and Wiz Magunda

2 Assessment and clinical risk 11
   Norman McClelland

3 Treatment approaches 21

   3.1 Introduction to treatment approaches 21
   Lorraine Conlon
   3.2 Relatives and carers 21
   Belinda Gasson
   3.3 Inter-professional working 28
   Rebecca Hills
   3.4 Vocational rehabilitation 31
   Rebecca Hills
   3.5 A psychoeducation model for schizophrenia 34
   Stuart Wix
   3.6 Therapeutic dilemmas in forensic practice 39
   Martin Humphreys and Norman McClelland

4 Dealing with hostility 42
   Mark West and Dave Abolins

5 Suicide/self-harm 73
   Shelly Allen and Sarah Beasley

6   Legal aspects   97
     Martin Humphreys, Emmanuel Oppong-Gyapong and Dave Mason

7   Education and training   105
     Norman McClelland and Joe Cutler

8   Diversion from custody   113
     Stuart Wix and Hayley Cushing

9   Aftercare   127
     Richard Carter, Gina Hillis and Andy Hunt

10   Future challenges   138
     Norman McClelland, Martin Humphreys and Lorraine Conlon

Index   141

List of contributors

Dave Abolins
Unit Manager, Reaside Clinic, Birmingham

Shelly Allen
Lecturer/Practitioner, Salford University, and Liaison Nurse/Crisis, Hope Hospital, Manchester

Sarah Beasley
Unit Manager, Reaside Clinic, Birmingham

Richard Carter
Forensic Community Psychiatric Nurse, Reaside Clinic, Birmingham

Lorraine Conlon
Head of Professional Nursing, Reaside Clinic, Birmingham

Hayley Ann Cushing
Forensic Community Psychiatric Nurse, Reaside Clinic, Birmingham

Joe Cutler
Staff Development Officer, Reaside Clinic, Birmingham

Belinda Gasson
Unit Manager, Reaside Clinic, Birmingham

Gina Hillis
Community Forensic Psychiatric Nurse, Ealing, Hammersmith and Fulham NHS Trust, Southall, Middlesex

Rebecca Hills
Head Occupational Therapist, Bracton Centre, Bexley; formerly Head Occupational Therapist, Reaside Clinic, Birmingham

Martin Humphreys
Senior Lecturer in Forensic Psychiatry, University of Birmingham and Reaside Clinic, Birmingham

Andy Hunt
Senior Social Worker, Reaside Clinic, Birmingham

Alex Kearns
Assistant Unit Manager, Reaside Clinic, Birmingham

Norman McClelland
Associate Director of Nursing, Tees and North East Yorkshire NHS Trust; formerly Lecturer in Forensic Nursing, University of Birmingham and Reaside Clinic

Wiz Magunda
Assistant Head of Nursing, Reaside Clinic, Birmingham

David Mason
Assistant Unit Manager, Reaside Clinic, Birmingham

Emmanuel Oppong-Gyapong
Unit Manager, Reaside Clinic, Birmingham

Phil Walsh
Unit Manager, Reaside Clinic, Birmingham

Mark West
Clinical Nurse Specialist, Reaside Clinic, Birmingham

Stuart Wix
Forensic Community Psychiatric Nurse and Team Leader, Reaside Clinic, Birmingham

Acknowledgements

We would like to acknowledge the help of all at Butterworth-Heinemann for their encouragement and support during the course of the production of this book. Thanks also to Gwen Robertson, Wendy Shannon and Susannah Busby. We are particularly grateful to Julie Busk for her tireless and patient efforts on our behalf in drafting and re-drafting each and every chapter of the book, acting as secretary to the editors and generally co-ordinating all our efforts.

NMcC
MH
LC
Birmingham 2001

Foreword

Nurses working within secure psychiatric services spend more time with mentally disordered in-patients than any other member of the multi-disciplinary team. They need to acquire diverse skills to enable them to provide effective care for some of the most difficult, disturbed and disadvantaged patients. Their unique relationship with the individual, their observations and ongoing assessments, are key to patient management and treatment.

This book distills the essence of best practice in forensic nursing from practitioners with many years' experience at Reaside Clinic. This is a medium secure unit within the West Midlands region. Its national reputation as a centre of excellence is, to a large measure, a reflection of the consistently high quality of nursing care provided there.

Within secure psychiatric settings there is a need to achieve a balance between therapeutic intervention and security. We get this wrong at our peril, as various inquiries have shown. A safe, therapeutic environment for patients, staff and visitors is the ultimate aim. Of crucial importance in achieving this is the attitude of nursing staff towards their patients in particular, and their wider role in general. This shapes the therapeutic environment and culture of a secure unit probably more than any other factor. Respect, tolerance and non-judgemental attitudes are needed. The chapters in this volume reflect these cultural values. They describe a continuum of care from initial assessment, through in-patient treatment to aftercare in the community. Throughout there is an emphasis on practical issues, grounded in a sound theoretical framework. How assessments are carried out, what information should be sought and the early planning of specific management strategies are thoroughly covered. There is a discussion of the importance of multi-professional team working for those caring for mentally disordered forensic patients. Examples of therapeutic interventions within secure environments are given substance, including specific rehabilitation programmes, a psycho-education model for those suffering from schizophrenia, and the involvement of relatives and carers. Other important themes covered include the practicalities of dealing with aggression and hostility as well as self-harming behaviours. The special skills and techniques required are described with the emphasis rightly placed on prediction, prevention and de-escalation.

Over the past decade as forensic practice has developed, the role of forensic nursing has also evolved, notably in relation to the wider community as well as in in-patient care. Forensic nurses have become involved in court diversion and liaison schemes. They frequently act as key workers under the Care Programme Approach and help to maintain difficult patients in the community. They must know about the Mental Health Act and relevant criminal legislation. Training, education and research by forensic nursing practitioners are vital in this field. All these areas are covered from a practical perspective, together with a glimpse into the future.

Finally, I wish to acknowledge the major contribution to and under-pinning of the practice described in this book by Tony Hillis, OBE. Tony was formerly Director of Nursing and Operational Manager at Reaside Clinic. He was one of the co-editors of this book, but very sadly died during the early stages of its production. He would have been very satisfied with this publication.

Rosemarie Cope
Clinical Director, Reaside Clinic

Introduction

Gina Hillis

When Tony Hillis visited the site in Birmingham where Reaside Clinic was to be built, his vision of what many now consider to be a centre of excellence in medium secure psychiatric care began to become a reality. He had worked extensively in nursing, in both England and abroad, and welcomed the challenge of his new post as Director of Nursing Services at Reaside Clinic. Tony's vision was one of a building that was at once comfortable and homely, but also encompassed some quite radical concepts of how to deliver high quality care in such a setting. Along with a commissioning team, Tony encouraged a philosophy of care which acknowledged that users of the services would, within the constraints of the law and clinical needs, have the same liberty, rights, autonomy and choice as any others while respecting the wishes of the wider community.

Tony was a person who naturally aspired to the teachings of Charles Handy, and embraced change, as it occurred in forensic practice, and within health care generally. The early years at Reaside Clinic were focused times, examining staff attitudes, building clinical teams, formulating new policies, and above all ensuring that the human rights and needs of mentally disordered offenders were met. Tony never ignored good practice in other areas, encouraging clinicians to travel throughout the UK and Europe. He promoted new service development, such as Court, Prison, and Police Station diversion schemes, bail hostel provision, as well as many varied educational and training programmes. Tony's commitment to the progression of forensic psychiatric nursing led to his founding the Forensic Psychiatric Nurses Association (FPNA), and remaining as Chairman until his untimely death in 1999. Tony recognised the importance of debate and dissemination of good practice and initiated an association newsletter, which led to the development of the journal *Psychiatric Care*, now *The British Journal of Forensic Practice*. He recognised the importance of sharing information and developing knowledge, and encouraged and supported the development of a very strong forensic academic base in the West Midlands. He negotiated academic posts with local universities, and supported, advised and taught on courses ranging from those developed in conjunction with the English National Board, to those provided at Masters level.

Tony's final career move was to Ealing, Hammersmith and Fulham NHS Trust, the territory of John Connolly, who before Tony had espoused the same sentiment of libertarianism in mental health care. Both aspired to least restrictive options, holistic care and held strong views about the use of seclusion. As had Connolly, Tony encouraged a non-judgemental attitude, as well as affording those unfortunate enough to become entangled in mental health and criminal justice services, dignity and respect. In the same way that Connolly contributed to the knowledge base in the Croonian Lectures, so too did Tony in his desire to contribute to the writing of this book.

Tony's overall contribution to nursing was recognised when he was awarded the OBE. His humility, however, would not allow him to accept it without claiming that it was for his colleagues and friends, and not solely himself. Many of his colleagues from the different professions who were fortunate to have worked alongside him have also remarked that he has made a significant contribution to their development, which has enabled them to translate this to benefit other services.

This book is a reflection of practice within Reaside Clinic, and more generally of evidence-based nursing in the UK currently. It is founded upon experience of forensic practice in one part of the West Midlands. This comes from a range of professionals' working practice as well as forensic mental health nursing. The three aspects of care as delivered by a medium secure unit, pre-admission assessment, in-patient care and care following discharge, are all examined within the book.

Forensic practice is unique in health care, in the relationship it has with the criminal justice system, some specific forms of assessment, working environment and provision of treatment, for those who present with a range of challenges. The preparation of nursing staff, and other professionals, to work in this area has led to specialist educational and training developments. These, as well as many other issues, are addressed here.

Referral to admission

Phil Walsh, Alex Kearns and Wiz Magunda

This chapter aims to give an understanding of the referral process and its structure. It involves discussion of the framework around which an admission unit should be resourced and managed.

The assessment and referral process is perhaps the key to effective intervention. Whyte and Youhill (1984) have described patient assessment as the collection and documentation of both primary and secondary information. McMurran and Hodge (1994) suggest that assessment is the most important step in trying to address maladaptive behaviours. They continue by stressing the importance of an accurate collection of data and its intelligent interpretation based on the patient's current health and past history, and how the patient has dealt with this. The assessment process described in this chapter includes a third dimension: that is, whether the patient's needs can be met by a service. If done correctly, assessment will provide information that will be used to plan the management of the patient, thus saving both time and resource. A poor assessment is likely to result in inappropriate admission, and delay in planning care. In certain circumstances a diverse patient mix with inappropriately placed patients will cause problems for the service (Higgins *et al.*, 1999). Such circumstances may create a situation where beds are blocked, and patient management becomes difficult at ward level.

Referrals to a medium secure psychiatric setting come from many sources:

- Prison doctor
- Solicitor
- Generic psychiatrist
- Special hospital
- Police
- Self-referral

A management team within a secure setting will have decided upon what service will be delivered and how this can be done. For example, the team may wish to operate a system for providing advice on care and management as well as specifically admitting individuals. The service may operate a Diversion At Point of Arrest scheme (DAPA). The full range of possibilities are discussed by Prins (1995).

Prison, general adult and other services will provide either urgent or routine referrals. Urgent referrals will generally mean that there is an immediate perceived risk. This may be toward others, in someone who is very assaultative, or someone who is wishing to leave and making determined efforts to do so. The risk may be to self, through refusing to eat or drink, or from intent or actions to self-harm. The routine referral is more likely to be made after discussion by the referrers who may have ongoing concerns about an individual, who may require care in a more secure environment.

A level of competence, as well as resourcefulness and an assertive nature, will be required to conduct an assessment. It is worth considering what the referring individual or team require, as in many cases management advice or treatment advice may be sufficient. Any advice given should be constructive and realistic, and where a patient is not to be transferred, it may be necessary to provide follow-up and support. Assessment also allows, for those who are to be admitted, a first point of contact with nursing staff from the unit where he/she may be later admitted.

The composition of the assessment/referral team should suit the specific needs of the patient. There may be core management or treatment issues that necessitate medical or nursing staff involvement; however, it is always necessary to engage the wider multi-professional team in the assessment process, either in discussion or via direct patient contact. This may occur where very specific interventions and needs are anticipated, and more thorough assessment and more robust discussion is required. Students from all disciplines may accompany staff on a referral assessment, and this should be recognised as a vital part of training, providing greater insight into forensic practice. When planning a referral assessment of a patient previously known to the service, consideration should be given to include within the assessing team a clinician who has had a positive rapport with the patient. This can contribute to the establishment of the relationship necessary for effective interview. The process by which the referral is received and subsequently assessed can be seen in Figure 1.1.

Following the assessment, the clinical team will discuss and further explore issues raised within the assessment interview, and actions recommended by the assessors. Before looking in detail at how the various stages of the process proceed we need to have an understanding of what information is required. At the end of the assessment there should be enough information to allow an informal discussion of the relevant issues to be addressed, and a decision to be made as to how to proceed. When looking at the information contained within a referral letter, it is worth remembering that information needs to be gleaned from all sources and not just at interview. The material taken from other reports should be cross-referenced at interview.

Developmental history

A developmental history needs to be addressed so as to gain an understanding of who the individual is and what their relationships are

Arrival
(phone/fax/mail)

Determination of specific needs

Referral Assessment Team

Assess urgency   Discussion

Arrange visit   Joint/team assessment?

Interview

Complete report

Clinical Team

Discussion to determine suitability for admission

Reassess?	Admit	Do not admit
Increase range of professional involvement	Bed Manager involvement	Inform referring team
	Maintain contact	Provide advice
	Arrange bed	
		Maintain contact
	Liaise with team	
	Ensure appropriate placement	

Figure 1.1

like with others. Examination of significant life events from birth is a useful approach. The following areas should be examined:

- Family relationships
- Progress in reaching childhood milestones (walking, talking etc.)
- School performance, and relationships with teachers and peers
- Use of illicit substances and alcohol
- Personal relationships (sexual development, sexual relationships, marital history)
- Family history (mental health, use of drugs, substances and alcohol, criminal activity and relationship with parents/siblings)
- Psychiatric history
- Physical health (past and current history, major accidents, head injuries etc.)
- Employment history

Criminal history

An understanding and review of previous offending and criminal history is also necessary. Many patients in secure units are referred because they may be presenting as a management problem in surroundings of lesser security. When referred, if individuals have no history of offending behaviour, then this is still worth documenting. A full list of offences should be recorded, inclusive of dates, sentencing, as well as a description which allows them to be put into context.

The index offence, or most immediate offence, should be documented, including details and antecedents and the individual's version of the offence, as well as their view of charges alleged, or sentence received.

Psychiatric history

As with the criminal history, there may be occasions when an individual has no psychiatric history. This fact will require documenting. In the event that an individual has a documented history, the following will need to be considered:

- History of admissions (dates/status/hospitals)
- Diagnoses
- Presenting behaviour during admission
- History of aggression (level of violence, antecedents, consequences)
- Attitude and insight to own criminal and psychiatric history
- Symptomatology and early warning signs
- Attempts at self injurious behaviour/suicide
- Absconding history
- Interventions, and their efficacy
- Current symptoms and management
- Medication history and compliance

Interview with patient

During an interview assessors should make note of, and later document, standard information regarding an individual's presentation and appearance:

- Personal hygiene
- Clothing (and relation to environment, temperature etc.)
- Physical manifestation of mood
- Psychomotor activity
- Any distinguishing physical features
- Visible evidence of self-harm

The interview itself may be formal or informal. A less formal approach may be needed, however, in order to attempt to get to know the individual. A conversational style is a useful one to adopt, with an acknowledgement of the importance of building a relationship before tackling what will be sensitive issues. The individual practitioner will assess which style is best for which situation. The following are worthy of consideration in such interview procedures:

- Current thoughts and feelings
- Sleep pattern, self care and nutrition
- Life history
- Insight/attitude to offence
- Speech
- Orientation
- Mood
- Individuals concerns

It is most important to differentiate, within any assessment documentation, the difference between factual data taken from the clinical record and the patient's/clinician's opinion or interpretation of events. The interview, and process of information gathering, are summarised in Table 1.1.

The stages outlined in Table 1.1 are largely self-explanatory. The pre-visit stage is used as the foundation for the rest of the process. Documentation at this stage will include a referral letter. This would ideally contain patient history as well as a description of the problem. Recent reports, such as updated admission summaries, may also be sent along with the initial referral. For individuals previously known to the service there will be data maintained in medical records. As well as examining available data, it is also worth noting what data may be missing, for instance a full list of previous offences and current charges may be vital. Those coming from other hospitals may not be subject to current court action, but details of any previous convictions are still important. For those charged with offences, or with previous criminal history, depositions will need to be seen. By this time, one may already be overwhelmed by the amount of information, but careful management will prevent this. Time should be afforded this process, which requires a review of all notes, prison or hospital. Using minutes of case conferences/clinical team meetings and examining incident forms in more detail, will provide a good overview, and direct an interviewer's attention to specific entries for specific days. Medication cards should be scrutinised to determine progression of treatment as well as compliance. Such information as is contained in these records may be of use in the future management of the patient. When there are problems associated with compliance for instance, thought may be given to the use of a liquid preparation or times of the day considered more favourable by the patient.

Table 1.1 Process of data collection

1. Pre-visit
- Examine documentation
- Assess completeness of data
- Establish issues of discussion pre-interview
- Establish issues of discussion for interview

2. Pre-interview
- Examine other documentation
- Assess completeness of data
- Discuss with staff
- Examine issues established at pre-visit stage

3. Interview
- Discuss care with patient
- Assess suitability for admission
- Examine issues set at pre-visit and pre-interview
- Establish post interview issues requiring clarification

4. Post interview
- Discuss with staff
- Assess completeness of data
- Examine content of interview
- Clarify any ambiguity

5. Clinical management discussion
- Discuss with other assessors
- Review all data
- Discuss further actions and recommendations with clinical team
- Clinical team decision

Incidents should be discussed with both the staff and later with the patient. Again, a critical eye will identify omission as well as inclusion in such accounts. The staff of the referring unit should be involved in a discussion of what the problems have been and what their concerns are. A non-threatening evaluation of current management, including direction of care, should also take place.

A multidisciplinary team interview will require planning, to determine the level and degree of structure, the order in which questions will be asked, and what questions to focus upon. This is necessary to avoid too much overlap.

Issues of safety and security should be addressed. Such issues should be discussed with staff on the referring unit. The assessing team will have familiarised themselves with methods of summoning assistance, as well as making themselves familiar with other alarms that may sound during the interview procedure. Staff presence (referring staff) during interview should be kept to a minimum so as to facilitate open discussion. At all times potential risk, to all those concerned, must be assessed and evaluated.

During an interview the individual should be given time to raise issues and questions of their own. This necessary process should be facilitated, but the focus and purpose of the interview should not be lost. It is important to clarify issues raised at both the pre-interview and pre-visit stages. Any immediate advice offered to a referring team will include perspectives from each professional on the assessing team. From nursing this may involve advice on management, observation levels, escorts and therapy/activity which may be useful. All comments ought to be constructive and realistic. The opportunity should be given to the referring team to discuss any recommendations, and the process of re-referral, should a situation deteriorate further.

Reasons for declining admission

If a patient can be safely managed with increased resources, e.g. special observations, then this may be possible without necessitating transfer. Accessing a bed within a secure setting because of such constraints may be inappropriate. There may also be occasions when the lack of a broad range of professionals in a referring team gives rise to a referral. Again, an assessing team needs to establish with service managers exactly what constitutes safe and effective care and treatment for patients. The following case study illustrates this well.

Case Study 1

An elderly man was referred due to a history of wandering off the ward. He had a diagnosis of schizophrenia with a psychiatric history going back thirty-five years. He was always agreeable to return but there had been recent instances of him not being found for periods of up to two days. His deteriorating eyesight gave rise to staff being concerned of harm from busy traffic etc. The referral letter mentioned three occasions of his being convicted of being drunk and disorderly, with a suggestion of him requiring a locked ward for his own safety.

The discussion concerning such a referral may give rise to a telephone discussion with the referral team, as opposed to sending an assessing team out. Advice would revolve around more appropriate placement within the referring hospital, a ward where a level of support exists, with a degree of security to prevent wandering and maintaining a care regime with a high level of observation.

A case example (Case Study 2) involving referral from a special hospital to a hospital of lesser security is illustrative of offending behaviour requiring more in-depth investigation.

Case Study 2

A female patient with a history of harming children is referred to Lower Security with a view to a period of trial leave. The referral letter reflects a number of trial community leave trips which have gone well. Examination of her clinical notes reveals no incident forms and no indication of problems. There is also no indication of her offending behaviour having been addressed, and no psychological reports of any depth. The patient's rationale for wanting to move relate to the fact that she has heard that special hospitals may close, and she is worried that bed blocking may occur in lesser secure environments. It is suggested that she be re-referred in the future once offending behaviour has been addressed.

Admission/the therapeutic environment

There are many visible components within the forensic psychiatric hospital setting which are clear evidence of an emphasis on safety and security, of patients, visitors, and staff. These manifest as common restrictions, peculiar to such environments, but differing between medium, maximum, and interim, or low secure environments. This work will not address specific differences, but will draw the reader's attention to the commonalties such as:

- Alarms (personal)
- An air lock (or double door)
- Anti-absconding systems in place on low level roof
- Keys
- A reception area monitoring movements
- A tannoy alarm or announcement system
- Observation windows
- Visitors being escorted
- Patients being escorted
- Controlled movements of some patients within and without the confines of the hospital

However, despite the above, the more modern purpose built unit will have many such measures built into the fabric and design of the building, minimising the obtrusive nature of such necessary measures. Such measures are designed so as to contribute to the supervision, management and safety of all. Such measures also contribute greatly to a continual assessment of risk. The NHS Estates (1993) document indicates the guidelines related to environments in which acute forensic care takes place. A basic feature of design is the degree of containment and subsequent effective management this affords. However, measures can be undertaken to reduce the 'custodial feel' of such buildings by adoption of courtyards surrounded by buildings, thus reducing the need for secure fences. A balance between security and domesticity is essential.

A combination of a safe environment and a homely atmosphere is the real focus of provision. Where a unit operates with more than one admission ward, then this provides ample opportunity to have differing, graduated levels of security, supervision, and a greater degree of provision of care according to specific needs. This can maximise individualised care programmes, and avoid patients requiring a high level of observation, becoming too institutionalised.

Staffing and admission

Staffing and skill mix is important when considering admitting patients to secure environments. Associated factors related to expected degree of clinical activity, staff confidence, experience and availability, as well as staff anxiety, are all linked to the success, or not, of an admission procedure.

Because of the sometimes unexpected nature of admissions to such units, it is usual for a degree of liberty to be afforded staffing levels on admission wards. The anticipated degree of activity level associated with an admission needs consideration when determining staff levels, as does the timing of the admission. The use of staff from other neighbouring wards may be appropriate to address staff numbers at times of high clinical/general activity. However, the domino effect, of borrowing staff, upon rehabilitation activities of other units should not be underestimated, hence it is worth avoiding such practices on a regular basis.

A confident, skilled and knowledgeable staff group is key to effective admission in secure environments. Clinical supervision will increase self-awareness, enabling clinicians to target areas for improvement on a regular basis. Managers who maintain levels of direct clinical activity, will, at once, ensure an effective understanding of clinical situations, and maintain a degree of respect and credibility.

The role of the multidisciplinary team is vital in ensuring that contact with the outside world is maintained during admission. The team can ensure that social networks are maintained, avoiding circles of isolation which may cause a patient to, in turn, increase isolative behaviours and non-co-operation during admission (Smith and McClelland, 1998). It is contact with the family at this time which is considered vital to settling a patient into an unfamiliar and potentially frightening environment. In the absence of the family and following referral from prison, the team will liaise with agencies such as probation and social services.

Conclusion

This is far from the conclusion, but rather the beginning of the in-patient care and assessment process. The referral and admission process will have provided a strong springboard to further assessment and the development of a holistic care package. The authors' experience reflects what may sometimes be a long settling in process. Patients who have been admitted from more secure hospital environments, or prisons, will test boundaries. This is to be expected; however, the use of 'blanket policies' relating to over-use of security, should be avoided. A continual process of clinical risk assessment developed at this stage will promote the individualised care reflected in the rest of this text.

References

Higgins, R., Hurst, K. and Wistow, G. (1999) Nursing acute psychiatric patients: a quantative and qualitative study. *Journal of Advanced Nursing*, 29 (January), pp. 52–63.

McMurran, M. and Hodge, J. (1994) *Assessment of Criminal Behaviours of Clients in Secure Settings*. Kingsley, London.

NHS Estates (1993) *Design Guide: Medium Secure Psychiatric Units*. NHS Estates, London.

Prins, H. (1995) *Offenders, Deviants or Patients?* Routledge, London.

Smith, N. and McClelland, N. (1998) Maintaining social networks. *Nursing Standard*, 25 March, Vol. 12, No. 27.

Whyte, L. and Youhill, G. (1984) The nursing process in the care of the mentally ill. *Nursing Times*, 80 (5), pp. 49–51.

Assessment and clinical risk

Norman McClelland

Introduction

Assessment revolves around the collection of data. The process will inform and guide future intervention(s) and evaluation of care delivered by nursing staff in their work with both the patient and the multiprofessional team. The mental health nurse will use a variety of methods to obtain information about the patient's physical, psychological and social states, in both past and present. Mental health nurses will use their knowledge of mental disorder, models of communication, psychological and physiological measurement, cultural variables, models of behaviour as well as sociology in their assessment of a patient's condition. This chapter will provide a brief overview of the principles of mental health nursing assessment; and illustrate how the role and working environment of forensic mental health nurses makes for differences between forensic nursing assessment and generic mental health nursing assessment. It will also describe the concept of risk assessment as an example of this difference.

The forensic mental health nurse (FMHN) will assess individuals in a wide variety of settings. These are not always conducive to making the best assessment, and do not represent what could be considered the best set of circumstances. An ideal environment is often described as a quiet unthreatening area, where a patient may feel at ease, is comfortable and can think and hear the questions being asked of them. The FMHN will often have to see individuals in places such as prisons, police cells, waiting and interview rooms in courts, in homeless shelters, and hospital wards which may be crowded and noisy. The individual being assessed may have to be escorted by prison officers, may be interviewed whilst being restricted in their movements, may be anxious because of their personal circumstances, or may be aggressive or violent during the interview. The criteria for referral to a medium secure or maximum secure psychiatric setting, revolve around clinical features in the case of particular patients which may have made them difficult to manage in the community or in a generic psychiatric setting, as well as requiring a greater degree of security than that which is already available. The transfer and/or restrictions placed upon individuals moved between hospitals and from prison to hospital are governed by the Mental Health Act 1983, and it is within the allied constraints and restrictions that the FMHN, in collaboration with multidisciplinary team members, must make his or her assessment.

The basic principles of assessment used in other areas of mental health nursing apply, but concepts associated with empathy and unconditional positive regard for example, may be more difficult to implement within a secure setting. Nursing students, and sometimes more experienced mental health nurses, may experience some difficulty in working with mentally disordered offenders due to the apparent lack of clarity about what constitutes mental disorder, and what is merely 'bad behaviour'. This, coupled with media sensationalised reporting of mental disorder and crime committed by the mentally unwell, can make this area of work unattractive to some. The constant bombardment of negative images from within the media, which is increasingly pervasive, could colour the attitudes of those clinicians planning to work in forensic practice. The end result may be confusion associated with assessment rationale and purpose in forensic psychiatric settings, allied with a tendency to be over-cautious.

Generic and forensic mental health nursing assessment

One way to avoid confusion in forensic practice is to retain and revisit the principles of assessment as they apply to all mental health settings, but make adaptations according to the needs of the environment and/or individual. Milne (1993), reviewing the approach required by mental health nurses during the assessment process, summarises the different dimensions in terms of direct and indirect methods. The basic rules of enquiry utilised in professions such as journalism are employed in Milne's description (see Box 2.1). These guidelines are important in recording assessment. It may be that in collating information the bulk of data comes from the notes or significant others because the individual being assessed does not wish to communicate, or is unable to, or does not see any benefit in talking to the assessing nurse. Milne (1993) makes reference to the triple response system dimension – thoughts, feelings and behaviour, or cognition, effect and responses. It is important that all of these areas are considered, but dependent upon circumstances, the assessment may necessarily be limited. Such limitations should be recorded as part of the assessment process.

In examining *why* there is a problem the responsibility of the FMHN is to review antecedents, consequences and behaviours associated with an incident(s). Care should be taken over referral assessments made to secure settings. Patients may be mismanaged, inappropriately placed, or even feared within the unit making the referral. The assessing FMHN, in collaboration with the clinical team, must make clear recommendations to the referring team, relating the reasons for accepting or rejecting the individual into secure care. The balance of security and therapy is such that the FMHN must establish and maintain the therapeutic relationship, be willing to take therapeutic risks, and engage in the monitoring and supervision deemed necessary, for instance, by the multidisciplinary team, the hospital or the Home Office.

Box 2.1 The dimensions of the assessment process

WHO   Who will provide the information?
           The assessor dimension

WHAT   What will be assessed?
           The triple response system dimension

WHY   Why is there a problem?
           The dimension from inside the patients to the relationship they
           have with others (level of assessment)

WHERE   Where will the assessment be conducted?
           The environmental dimension

WHEN   When will an assessment be conducted?
           The temporal dimension

HOW   How is the information to be gathered?
           The strategy dimension, which technique is best?
           The selection of an appropriate instrument

Source: Milne, 1993, p. 84

In forensic practice the basic principles of assessment apply, and it is likely that there will be use of interview, diary work, observation and record sheets, as well as psychosocial and psychometric assessment.

Group assessment, tends to be used less frequently in forensic mental health settings than perhaps elsewhere. The notion of individualised care or a problem solving approach as integral to the assessment process in forensic mental health practice is more predominant. One reason for this may be the unwillingness on the part of this patient group to share details of index offences. This, coupled with the need to focus on particular individual risk factors, requires the use of individualised assessments in forensic practice as opposed to a use of specific assessment packages. This is not to suggest that group methods such as those used in anger management group work are not useful. Indeed, some are used in forensic practice (see Novaco, 1994).

Nursing assessment tends not to be so well described as assessment undertaken by other professionals in the health field.

> In contrast to the psychiatric nurse other members of the multidisciplinary team such as Psychologists and Doctors have well defined categories of assessment. (Ritter, 1989, p. 4)

Ritter goes further in describing nursing assessment as 'heterogeneous', and how such an assessment must make sense to people other than the nurse and the patient. Thus the liaison the nurse has with other members of the team, the relationship that the nurse has with the patient, and the recording systems utilised by the nurse all begin to steer the assessment in a specific way. The systematic recording of data from the patient, and from other sources, prior to admission, is a vital part of the assessment process, as is the identification and measurement of specific behaviours to be assessed, a team process, shortly after admission. The focus of this approach may be the index offence, the immediacy of 'risk behaviour' presenting problems associated with self harm, violence, and/or aggression, mental state, severe self-neglect or the risk of exploitation. These are all areas usually associated with assessment of individuals referred to, or resident in secure psychiatric settings.

Risk assessment

Risk assessment may be viewed as the focus of assessment work by forensic mental health nurses (FMHN). Numerous authors recognise the importance of an objective systematised approach to assessing and predicting potentially dangerous behaviour (Scott, 1977; Pollock and Webster, 1990; McClelland, 1995a). One of the main difficulties associated with the assessment of risk is that the clinician is always aware that any prediction of risk can never be 100 per cent certain. However this should not detract from the recognition that there are factors which can be identified and examined, which inform an assessors picture of how patients may behave in future. The importance of risk assessment and the process involved is summarised by Gunn:

> The aim is to assess the factors which have led that patient to be aggressive, to ascertain how many of those factors are amenable to change, and then to intervene to alter the factors, so that risks of aggression are reduced. (Gunn, 1993, p. 633)

The importance of a process within psychosocial risk assessment is, as previously stated, extremely important. Barker suggested that:

> In assessment we begin to write the story of someone's life. (Barker, 1986, p. 55)

There are clear stages to the assessment. The first stage is the recording of a patient history. Major areas of difference in forensic assessment are in terms of the focus, and the amount of detail recorded in specific areas. Further to this, any process which takes place in a secure setting between a clinician and a client, who may be detained against their wishes, suggests an unequal relationship. However the FMHN should endeavour to apply the principles of assessment related to open and honest communication and a reaffirmation of why one is seeking specific items of information and a willingness to take into account all information offered. This again relates to the work of Milne (see Box 2.1).

The history will include and reflect a detailed criminal and psychiatric history, as well as information pertaining to the index offence. The nurse–patient relationship is established and improved through an informal discussion on admission which will detail the necessity of a range of informal interviews in the early part of admission for this purpose.

The FMHN, and other members of the clinical team, will have already begun a process whereby detail from previous clinical notes, school reports, police records, social and psychological enquiries as well as depositions related to previous offending and the index offence will have been recorded. Formal sessions with a client, following admission, establish a process of self-report. The nurse can make the choice of whether such interviews are structured or unstructured. However, there are clear advantages to examining, via specific questions, a range of variables related to previous violence, drug and alcohol use, personal relationships, employment and housing, specific interests (i.e. cruelty, racism sadism), factors related to the availability of victims, weapons, declared intentions and attitudes to victims and others, and mental state, particularly paranoia, anger and rage (see Gunn, 1993).

The index offence constitutes a part of the psychiatric and criminal history. It is key that the nurse records specific detail related to the offence or other relevant behaviour if an offence has not occurred. This would include the date of the offence, details of any known victim, where the offence occurred, and at what time. The majority of enquiry reports into forensic practice in the early 1990s relate that it is this latter information which was often missing from clinical case notes, leading clinicians to make ill-informed judgements about the potential risk an individual client presented in a given circumstance (see Peay, 1996). The recorded index offence information will be virtually the same data as previously recorded as client history and will reflect the areas outlined previously. The importance of third party information cannot be stressed enough. It is the responsibility of the nurse and the clinical team to arrange similar interviews with family and/or significant others to determine their opinions on the client's history, and events that led to the offence and/or admission. Thus the first stage of this risk assessment has begun to establish the potential for emergent patterns of behaviour between history (recorded, self-report, and third party) and the most recent behaviour which brought the client to the attention of the forensic service.

The second stage of the assessment in many ways reflects the FMHN's role as key worker. In terms of the nursing process it would appear that this is where assessment moves on to planning and implementation. However, the essence of this second stage of risk assessment is based around a series of planned interventions which in turn will lead to reassessment, as Ritter indicates:

Assessment is a dynamic activity, and occurs in at least five forms – on admission, in objective measurements, in interaction process recordings, in progress notes and in the evaluation of plans. (Ritter, 1989, p. 3)

The FMHN will therefore begin to develop specific plans of intervention which should revolve around determining which cognitive affective and situational factors predisposed individuals to offending behaviour which may include violence and/or aggression. McClelland (1995a) reflected on how important it was for the nurse to be aware of the work of individual team members. Such an awareness can assist the delivery of an holistic approach to assessment, in that a team approach should reflect the specific areas of expertise found among team members. It is at this stage of assessment that one could expect a range of interventions which may include psychometric and psychosocial assessment, the use of observation charts or rating scales, specific observation of patient behaviours, a further use of structured/unstructured interview and situational assessment in a combination of restricted and unrestricted environments. Running in parallel to all of the above, will be a monitoring and evaluation of any medication the client may or may not be prescribed, and consequent alteration in behaviour and/or mental state.

The nature of individualised client-focused care encourages the nurse to be both creative and innovative in their approach at this stage. The nurse should have built up a sufficient rapport and relationship with the patient to enable them to gather data on maladaptive behaviours related to violence, aggression, and anger. The FMHN will have encouraged the patient to engage in either one-to-one or group work related to anxiety and/or anger management. It may be the case in medium secure units that a patient's lack of control leads to their being a risk to themselves and/or others. It must be remembered that anger is not always a negative emotion, but can function as a useful control in itself. Within the framework of an anger management group there is scope for focus work concentrating on environmental, cognitive, affective and behavioural aspects for individual patients. There is also scope for self-report, the use of analogue scales, role play, anger diaries, and psychometric assessment. Novaco and Welsh (1989) have written extensively on the role that cognitive mediation plays in anger disturbance. McClelland (1995b) relates how an anger management group was formed in one secure unit for patients who displayed evidence of a difficulty in controlling anger, and who further expressed dissatisfaction in their own ability to deal with their anger, or provocation by others. Many of the methods described here were used in this group work, and some were also incorporated into care plans devised by the key worker at ward level. Thus, for example, patients could be observed in terms of their speech and behaviour in relation to anger both within the group setting and on an individual basis. Re-assessment occurred as a consequence of specific interventions conducted within the group.

Discussion amongst the multiprofessional facilitators, on completion of the work, revolved around the importance of integrating this sort of approach into care plans in a more detailed manner in future. The range of interventions carried out within this group led to detailed assessment of recognised determinants of anger such as environmental circumstances, physiological arousal and cognitive processes and structures. This in turn provided nurses working within the group, and on the ward, with a greater understanding of individual client's behavioural responses. McHugh *et al.* (1995), in describing a de-escalation model related to violence and aggression, spoke of a range of methods in assessing and managing such behaviour. They included problem solving, counselling, communication, autonomy and negotiation as key to their model. The de-escalation models of intervention, and the assessment processes inherent within these, should be at the core of FMHN intervention regarding violence and aggression. These same authors (McHugh *et al.*, 1995) related how the unmanaged escalation of anxiety in an inpatient setting can significantly unsettle a therapeutic environment. They also described a 'circle of therapeutic intervention' which encourages empowerment of a patient following an aggressive or violent incident leading to improved self-control.

The importance of documentation diaries/self-reports etc. to the assessment process cannot be over-stressed. The collection of such material in the final stages of a psychosocial risk assessment, and the presentation approach, which must clearly specify differences in factual data and nurses opinion, is also important. The opinion serves the function of analysis and prediction. This in itself is a different enough concept for many clinicians to accept – appraisal of probability, on the basis of behaviour observed in what may be described as an artificial environment. However, if the FMHN is clearly differentiating between factual recorded data and opinion, then the feasibility of future treatments or interventions to prevent or reduce violence or aggression in certain environments can be assessed. It is the responsibility of the assessing FMHN, in conjunction with the multi-disciplinary team, to identify salient points, pertaining to areas such as remorse, fluctuations in mental state, anger control, specific incidents of violence/aggression, as well as the patient's perception of such recorded assessment information.

The notion of objectivity in assessment relates to what Grounds (1995) has referred to as 'distinguishing between worry and risk'. He writes of how 'worry' and 'risk' are not well correlated.

We practise within a culture that could be accused of being inquiry-driven, and consequently reactive. The range and extent of inquiries into the care, treatment and management of the mentally ill during the 1990s was extensive. To be reactive, however, is not always to be negative. Inquiries can have significant impact upon clinical practice, which in turn focuses assessment priorities and reinforces the need for specific assessment. Prins (1993), in the inquiry into the death of Orville Blackwood, brought the need to assess reasons for secluding an individual, as well as administering medication and urgent treatment, sharply into focus. The Ritchie Inquiry (1994) into the care and treatment of Christopher Clunis contributed to changes in the way in which patients are supervised and managed in the community. We must learn to balance worry and concern with the reality of the presenting behaviour. Morgan (1998) reminds us of the importance of on-going assessment rather than hunches or gut reaction, and the necessity of ensuring a collaborative and empowering approach to risk assessment. Further to this, he reaffirms the importance of understanding the service users' experiences of risk, discussion revolving around potential for risk behaviour, and the importance of encouraging therapeutic risk-taking. Morgan's work relates to all practice, but the focus has been the community. Risk assessment is now closely linked to community care and places emphasis on an area that has received much criticism related to inadequate follow-up, poor liaison and communication, as well as inappropriate support provided to patients in the community.

Box 2.2 provides a case example of the assessment process. This should, of course, not be seen as a static, single process, but a dynamic evolving procedure which requires constant monitoring and reappraisal.

This chapter has focused largely on the psychosocial assessment of risk as an underpinning principle of assessment in forensic practice. There are many behaviours and mental disorders, seen in both generic and forensic

Box 2.2 A case study: Tommy

Tommy is a 38-year-old male, separated from his wife and three children, two of whom are experiencing behavioural problems at school related to violence and aggression. Tommy is reported as having a volatile nature, having behaved in aggressive and violent ways in the past to achieve respect from his wife and family. He is a known drug user, and has absconded from an extended period of leave in the community. Prior to his absconsion Tommy had been verbally aggressive three times in the previous 12 months.

Assessment

A holistic assessment of risk would incorporate key forensic elements such as violence/self harm–suicide/mental state/relationship with relatives/severe neglect/exploitation/and a summary examining immediate dangers and imminent risks presented by Tommy, as well as the potential for harm he may possess. A duty to warn would also be incorporated into the risk assessment.

Who — will provide information? Wife, family, children, nursing staff, friends, known associates. The focus of this area of assessment would revolve around the risk as perceived by those felt by the clinical team to be most at risk. Alternatively, those who are interviewed may believe Tommy to be at risk from others, and this can be incorporated into an assessment accordingly.

What — will be assessed? The thoughts, feelings, and behaviours of all concerned parties would also be incorporated into the assessment. The clinical team would reflect upon previous instances of absconsion by Tommy, and assess the chances of harm to self/others, the chance of illicit drug use, the time factor in terms of his return to hospital, and where he may have gone. It is at this early stage when consideration could be given as to how to manage Tommy on his return.

Why — is there a problem? What mood was Tommy in when he absconded? Why did he abscond? The clinical team must assess antecedent events to the absconsion, and what Tommy understands the consequences of such behaviour to be. The key worker will perhaps reflect upon this temporary breakdown in care, and further reflect upon possible outcomes of the overall process, with respect to whether to be more or less restrictive, and further analysis of eventual consequences of the behaviour.

Where and when — will assessment be conducted? It is likely that assessment will occur with family in their own home and/or hospital. Friends and family and associates are likely to be interviewed in the community. The assessment of Tommy himself will occur in a temporal dimension which spans his time prior to absconsion, reports of him during the absent period and following his return.

How — is information to be gathered? In this instance an antecedents, behaviour, consequences (ABC) analysis will have been useful to examining reasons for the absconding behaviour, and how better to communicate and manage such behaviour, should it occur in the future.

psychiatric hospital settings. However, some assessment tools have been developed for use primarily in secure settings. McKeown and McCann (1995) write of a schedule for assessing relatives for schizophrenia in a secure environment, and Woods (2000) described of the use of the Behavioural Status Index (BSI) in the social assessment of risk. One actuarial risk assessment, the Risk Assessment, Management, and Audit system (RAMAS; O'Rourke *et al.*, 1997) shows how an actuarial tool can offer a framework where risk assessment can lead to risk management strategies. These authors have suggested that this easy-to-use instrument, which incorporates needs and skills assessment, as well as suggested risk management strategies, helps all clinicians to measure four particular areas of risk:

1. Dangerousness
2. Mental instability
3. Self harm
4. Vulnerability

The assessment process would endeavour to ensure involvement of a range of clinicians, including the police and probation service. Patient participation is also integral to the assessment process. The quality checks inherent in the process relating to completeness of information, contributions of all, corroborated evidence, concerns and continuing care, are all part of the systematic approach.

Risk assessment in forensic practice requires the clinician to be aware of current developments, as well as the use of evidence based practice, and this in turn highlights the need for education and training as well as appropriate clinical supervision. Clinical assessment in secure psychiatric settings, as in many others, is heavily reliant upon detailed recording of information throughout, prior to direct contact, during admission and beyond.

References

Barker, P. (1986) Mechanical faults. Mental health nursing. *Nursing Times*, 82 (39), pp. 55–6.

Grounds, A. (1995) Risk assessment and management in clinical context. In John Crichton (ed.), *Psychiatric Patient Violence: Risk and Response*. Duckworth, London.

Gunn, J. (1993) Dangerousness. In J. Gunn and P.J. Taylor (eds) *Forensic, Psychiatric, Clinical, Legal and Ethical Issues*. Butterworth-Heinemann, Oxford, pp. 625–45.

McClelland, N. (1995a) The assessment of dangerousness: a procedure for predicting potentially dangerous behaviour. *Psychiatric Care*, 2 (1), pp. 17–20.

McClelland, N. (1995b) Look back at anger. *Nursing Times*, 8 February, Vol. 91, No. 6, pp. 59–61.

McHugh, A., Wain, I. and West, M. (1995) Handle with care. *Nursing Times*, 8 February, Vol. 91, No. 6, pp. 62–3.

McKeown, M. and McCann, G. (1995) A schedule for assessing relatives : the Relative Assessment Interview for schizophrenia in a secure environment. *Psychiatric Care*, 2 (3): 84–8.

Milne, D. (1993) Assessment. In *Psychology and Mental Health Nursing*. Macmillan, London. Section 2, pp. 49–81.

Morgan, S. (1998) The assessment and management of risk. In Charlie Brooker and Julie Repper (eds) *Serious Mental Health Problems in the Community: Policy, Practice and Research*. Balliere, Tindall, London, ch. 12.

Novaco, R.W. (1994) Anger as a risk factor for violence among the mentally disordered. In J. Monahan and Henry J. Steadman (eds), *Violence and Mental Disorder: Developments in Risk Assessment*. University of Chicago Press, London, pp. 21–61.

Novaco, R.W. and Welsh, W. (1989) Anger disturbances: cognitive mediation and clinical prescriptions. In: K. Howells and C. Hollin (eds) *Clinical Approaches to Violence*. John Wiley, London, pp. 39–60.

O'Rourke, M.M., Hammond, S.M. and Davies, E.J. (1997) Risk assessment and risk management: the way forward. *Psychiatric Care*, 4 (3), pp. 104–6.

Peay, J. (1996) *Inquiries after Homicide*. Duckworth and Company, London.

Pollock, N. and Webster, C. (1990) The clinical assessment of dangerousness. In R. Bluglass and P. Bowden (eds), *Principles and Practice of Forensic Psychiatry*. Section VII: *Violence*. Churchill Livingstone, Edinburgh.

Prins, H. (Chairman) (1993) 'Big Black and Dangerous?' Report of the Committee of Inquiry into the Death in Broadmoor Hospital of Orville Blackwood. S.H.S.A., London.

Ritchie, J.H. (Chairman), Dick, D. and Lingham, R. (1994) The Report of the Inquiry into the Care and Treatment of Christopher Clunis. HMSO, London.

Ritter, S. (1989) Nursing Assessment. In *Bethlem Royal and Maudsley Hospital Manual of Clinical Psychiatric Nursing Principles and Procedures*. Harper Row, London, ch. 1, pp. 3–11.

Scott, P.D. (1977) Assessing dangerousness in criminals. *British Journal of Psychiatry*, 131, 127–42.

Woods, P. (2000) Social assessment of risk: the Behavioural Status Index. In D. Mercer, T. Mason, M. McKeown and G. McCann (eds), *Forensic Mental Health Care: A Case Study Approach*. Churchill Livingstone, London, ch. 12, pp. 333–9.

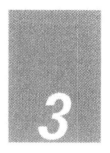

Treatment approaches

3.1 Introduction to treatment approaches

Lorraine Conlon

Therapy on an individual and group basis gives patients the opportunity to seek validation, give and receive interpersonal feedback and test new and different ways to improve their quality of life.

The nurse in the role of facilitator may function autonomously or in collaboration with other professionals. Effectiveness depends not on the facilitator's background discipline but rather on the match between the abilities and characteristics of the facilitator and the needs of the patients.

This chapter discusses three approaches of group and individual interventions with which nurses are involved and emphasises, in the last two sections of the chapter, issues around interpersonal working and therapeutic dilemmas faced by practitioners.

3.2 Relatives and carers

Belinda Gasson

A major criticism of institutional practice is that it removes the individual identified as the 'patient' from the family and social context in which their problems occur. As a result they may become divorced from key relationships and vital supports. While current community policies are advocated out of such concerns, for the mentally disordered offender the possibilities for bridging the divide can be extremely limited. This brings with it not only the stigma of mental illness but the added burden of criminality.

For families with a relative who is a patient of forensic psychiatric services these problems can be particularly important. The patient's liberty has been removed, for some without limit of time, and the ability of relatives and carers to maintain contact can be limited. This may be due to geographical distance or loss of economic structure causing both financial and domestic difficulties, as well as the psychological and emotional trauma experienced. The early stages of admission in particular may be problematic. Relatives or carers are often bewildered by the patient's symptoms. Even if they have

Box 3.1 Relatives and carers questionnaire

1 Please indicate which of the topics below you would be interested in hearing more about:

Resources and facilities at the Reaside Clinic
Welfare and Social Benefits
Medication
The Mental Health Act
Mental Health Tribunals
Rehabilitation and preparation for discharge
After care
Practical problems in caring for discharge

The above list represents some of the topics that could be considered in a Relatives Support Group. Please indicate below any areas of particular interest to you that could become a focus of discussion in such a group:

2 The care of patients at Reaside Clinic is organised multiprofessionally. It is hoped that representatives from each discipline will be contributing to the group discussions. Please indicate if there are particular disciplines you would like to be represented in one or more of the group discussions:

Psychiatrist
Psychologist
Nurse
Occupational Therapist
Social Worker
Community Psychiatric Nurse
Pharmacist

3 Would you find a Relatives Support Group beneficial?
YES   NO

4 How often would you like the group to meet?
Weekly
Fortnightly
Monthly
Other

5 How long do you think each meeting should last?
One hour
One and a half hours
Two hours
Other

6 What day and time would be most convenient for these meetings to be organised?
Weekdays
Weekends

Afternoons
Evenings

7 Please state your area of residence, i.e. the nearest town or village. *Do not give your address.*

8 Would attending such a group at the Reaside Clinic cause you any particular difficulties?
YES   NO
If Yes please specify

9 Have you any additional comments or suggestions? If Yes please detail them below.

Thank you for your cooperation in completing this form.

heard of schizophrenia, for example, they may have no idea what it means other than what they know as a result of media representation and reporting of mental illness. They may also be dealing with other experiences that are quite new to them, such as the complexities of institutions, legal issues, and the inevitable contact with a wide range of professionals involved.

For relatives and carers where the individual will, at some time in the future, return to, or visit the family home, there can be considerable concerns about re-accommodating the patient and managing his or her potentially undesirable behaviour. Some relatives and carers will also experience isolation and marginalisation as a result of the situation they find themselves in, isolated by their lack of understanding of the patient's mental health problems, and feeling distanced from the professionals involved in their care and treatment. Difficulties may be further compounded if the patient's index offence has occurred in the local community. It is not unusual if this has been the situation, for relatives and carers to be stigmatised and marginalised by those around them. There will also be a small group of relatives and carers who will have been the victim of the patient's aggression or violence. Given such situations it is understandable that relatives and carers may experience overwhelming emotions of anger, guilt or fear. Worrall (1990) highlights the importance of health professionals taking into account the overall impact of illness and disability in the social context of the family, suggesting that the focus of care and support should not rest exclusively with the individual who is ill. Relatives tend to request information, guidance and understanding rather than 'treatment'.

The fundamental part of patient care in forensic settings and beyond should therefore be to adopt a therapeutic approach to the care and support of relatives and carers. Staff should seek to expand the therapeutic potential of care. It should be acknowledged that relatives and carers have a significant role to play in supporting the patient and are integral to the patient's rehabilitation and eventual re-integration back into a community. It should be equally recognised that such relatives and carers have their own needs and difficulties that must be addressed if a truly holistic approach is to be achieved.

In a study at one regional secure unit all listed next of kin were sent questionnaires (see Box 3.1) about the need for some form of formal support structure. Forty per cent of questionnaires were returned, and 96 per cent of responders indicated that a Relative and Carer Support Group would be useful for them.

Once the survey information had been collated, all next of kin were invited to an informal meeting to share the survey findings and discuss how things should be moved forward. The first meeting was attended by eighteen relatives and carers. Apart from presenting the survey information the meeting provided an opportunity for other relatives and carers to meet with staff who would be involved in future groups. After the initial survey outcomes were presented, relatives, carers and staff divided into three small groups to informally discuss thoughts and ideas about the formation of a Relative and Carers Support Group. The discussions from these groups were then fed back into the meeting as a whole. Views were positive and participants were most forthcoming about what they required. This included information and education on a range of topics. Mullen and Bebbington (1992, p. 207) expressed the view that 'giving simple information to relatives about the nature and course of mental illness and about the provision of services may be easily overlooked by clinicians concerned with more esoteric aspects and management'. Relatives and carers also felt that it would be helpful to have contact with different professionals involved in the care of patients. They were to add that one of the most helpful aspects of the meeting had been the opportunity to exchange views and share experiences with others. It was subsequently agreed that a Relative and Carers Support Group would be established. Meetings would take place on the last Saturday of each month between 6.30 p.m. and 8 p.m. Reflecting on many of the concerns and issues outlined served as a catalyst for the exploration and eventual formation of a support network for relatives and carers.

There appeared little experience to draw on and scarce literature to review in relation to such a group in forensic psychiatric services. Tarrier *et al.* (1988) stress the need to ensure objective data collection from specific subject groups, in order to meet their concerns and offer the information required to the identified target group. To obtain the information required the questionnaire was based on questions raised by relatives and carers with staff previously. Many of the issues raised by relatives and carers in their discussions were of a practical nature. Examples of their concerns included financial issues, entitlements to benefits and lack of understanding about legal processes and procedures. Other issues were some of the difficulties they had organising visits. Women in particular who did not want to bring children to visits had difficulties arranging childcare. Those without their own transport expressed worries about using public means and travelling long distances in the hours of darkness. Elderly or disabled relatives and carers often needed to rely on others to bring them. Many had questions about the patient's illness, treatment and care. They also expressed concerns about the future in relation to the patient and their own ability to cope. Examples of such issues raised were:

- Tell me about the illness, what are the signs and symptoms?
- What medication are they taking, are there any side effects?
- Why is rehabilitation so important, what does it involve?
- What support is available in the community for the patient and myself?
- Whom do I contact if there is a crisis following discharge?
- What are the options for accommodation when discharged from hospital?
- Are there any employment or training schemes available for someone with mental health problems?

Not only did relatives and carers seek information on the nature of the patient's illness, treatment and future plans, but they often displayed a curiosity about the roles of different professionals involved in the various aspects of the patient's assessment, treatment and care. However, frequently underlying these discussions there was a sense of isolation which often related to the lack of opportunity to discuss and share their own particular problems as a relative or carer of someone with severe mental health problems.

The Relative and Carers Support Group

A group was established whose members were homogeneous and consisted of relatives and carers who provided support for the patient outside the institutional setting. The emphasis of the group was education, on topics defined by the members and delivered by professionals, and to encourage social interaction and an opportunity to share experiences and offer mutual support. Kuipers *et al.* (1992, p. 95) suggest that 'groups expand relatives' social networks which are often reduced by living with schizophrenia, they help relieve the resultant feelings of guilt and stigma'.

Aims and objectives of the support group

1. To provide education on topics that enabled relatives and carers to be better informed about mental health problems and mental health issues.
2. To facilitate contact with a wide group of professionals and non-professionals with knowledge or expertise in particular areas of mental health.
3. To encourage relatives and carers to offer suggestions of how services could be improved for themselves and patients.
4. To provide a supportive, safe environment where relatives and carers were able to interact socially and to share experiences and offer support.
5. To continue to offer support, minimise distress and reduce the stress or anxiety that relatives and carers may experience.

The group has tended to focus on a needs-led approach, rather than professional assumptions. Each meeting opens with individual relatives and carers introducing themselves and giving a brief background of why they are there and what they hope to gain from the experience. This is followed by a short presentation on a topic related to mental health, with time for questions and discussion. The latter part of the meeting is given over to interactions between group members. This frequently involves individuals sharing their personal perspectives and experiences of being a carer of someone with mental health and associated problems.

Concepts of the group

The framework underpinning the processes, dynamics and culture of the group are based on concepts Yalom (1985) defines as 'therapeutic factors'. These are based on an interpersonal approach rather than a psycho-analytical one, and include:

1. Instillation of hope.
2. Universality.
3. Imparting information.
4. Altruism.
5. Re-capsulation of the family experience.
6. Social learning.
7. Initiative behaviour.
8. Interpersonal learning.
9. Cohesiveness.
10. Catharsis.
11. Existential factors.

Instillation of hope
This has been vital. The opportunity to observe and interact with others, who have experienced similar problems and have adopted a more positive and optimistic view of the future and their situation, can give hope and have significant impact on those still struggling to come to terms with issues.

Universality
The discovery that individuals are not alone in their problems and difficulties can reduce the sense of isolation: 'The sense of uniqueness is heightened by social isolation' (Yalom (1985, p. 7).

Imparting information
This has been relevant to the educational component of the group and including the sharing of information between relatives and carers.

Altruism
By sharing experiences and learning that individuals have something to offer others carers can begin to value themselves.

Cohesiveness
This has been important to the group, from identifying the concept of

belonging to and being accepted as a valued member of a group that works collectively to alleviate or resolve difficulties. Kuipers *et al.* (1992, p. 95) advocate 'that a wider variety of solutions to difficult problems are likely to be proposed by a group rather than a family which may contain only one relative'.

Catharsis

Relatives and carers are able to share experiences and express feelings in an environment where they feel others will be empathic, in that they will have had similar experiences and therefore will be able to identify with the situation.

The interventions used by therapists facilitating the group have been based on the fundamental principles and core conditions of a counselling approach. This has included using techniques of building rapport, facilitating trust, warmth and empathy, through a process of active listening, reflecting, questioning, clarifying and summarising. Staff involved have come from a variety of professional backgrounds including nursing, occupational therapy and social work. Other professional groups have contributed in making educational presentations.

The future of the group

The group described here has been established for six years and significant change has taken place since it commenced. In line with current policy and legislation, multiprofessional teams have adopted an individual approach which aims to ensure that relatives and carers receive the support and information they require. As a result there has been a reduction in the demand for educational topics, and generally relatives and carers feel their needs are now being met more on an individual level. The group continues to meet monthly as a Relative and Carers Forum.

Many positive developments have evolved. A library of videos, books and information leaflets is available for relatives and carers, and an information booklet has been produced. A directory of organisations and telephone numbers of services that will provide support, information and advice for relatives and carers available in the local community has been published.

The aim of the group has been to enable and empower, by engaging members in a therapeutic process that aims to acknowledge their problems and difficulties, but primarily to validate their roles as carers. As Beck (1999, p. 47) has said, 'relatives and carers are the stakeholder of care in the community and professionals must be encouraged to work with them and for them'.

References

Beck, R. (1999) Support for the carers of people with schizophrenia. *Nursing Times*, 95 (2), pp. 46–7.

Kuipers, L., Leff, J. and Lamm, D. (1992) *Family Work for Schizophrenia*. Royal College of Psychiatrists, London.

Mullen, R. and Bebbington, P.E. (1992) A workshop for relatives of people with chronic mental illness. *Psychiatric Bulletin*, 16 (4), pp. 206–7.

Tarrier, N., Barrowclough, C., Vaugn, C. Bamrah, J. S., Porceddu, K., Watts, S. and Freeman, C. (1988) The community management of schizophrenia. A controlled trial of a behavioural intervention with families to reduce relapse. *British Journal of Psychiatry*, 153, pp. 532–42.

Worrall, G.P. (1988) In J. Wilson (ed.) *Self Help Groups*. Longman Group, Essex.

Yalom, I.D. (1985) *Theory and Practice of Group Psychotherapy*, 3rd edn. Basic Books, New York.

3.3 Inter-professional working

Rebecca Hills

It is common practice for much in health care to be provided by a 'team' of some kind, and whether multidisciplinary or primary health care, the fundamental desire for professionals to work together remains the same. As the care of patients with mental health problems has resulted in some well publicised and adverse incidents so the profile of health professionals has been raised to a level where constant scrutiny by the public has become a fact of life. Increasingly generic mental health teams look to forensic services for advice on the management of difficult or dangerous patients (Friel and Chaloner, 1996), and for forensic mental health professionals to work collaboratively with both mainstream providers of mental health and other agencies (Shepherd, 1995). The development of inter-professional team working is believed to have developed within health services for a number of reasons. The pressure to establish an integrated approach to care has evolved partly as a result of the many child abuse scandals and mental health related tragedies. There has also been an increasing conviction that inter-professional work is a more cost-effective means of providing care (Rawson, 1994). Kane (1980) believes that teamwork developed initially within social work in response to a lack of power. This led to interest from all professional, primarily nursing, pharmacy and occupation therapy and, latterly, the medical profession. In contrast, Barr and Waterton (1994) describe the need for collaboration having been the result of government reforms in health and social care and therefore more a response to a directive than an altruistic desire to improve the situation.

This section will review the advantages of inter-professional working in the provision of forensic mental health services, the potential difficulties that may arise and issues related to communication and collaboration.

Inter-professional team working: the advantages and the difficulties

The health team has been defined as a 'group who share a common health goal and common objectives, determined by community needs, to the achievement of which each member of the team contributes, in accordance with his or her competence and skill and in co-ordination with the functions of others' (WHO, 1984, p. 13). This somewhat unwieldy definition does have the advantage that it summarises both the method and function of an inter-professional team effectively.

Health care professionals work in teams for a number of reasons. McGrath (1991) describes two central themes, these being increased effectiveness in service provision and the creation of a more satisfying working environment. However, teams also produce an holistic approach to client care, allow systems to be tackled, encourage overall service planning and encourage preventative work. The need to ensure effective service provision within forensic mental health and the potential results of not doing so are clear from a brief review of the numerous Public Inquiry reports into incidents involving mental health patients over recent years. The environments in which forensic mental health services are provided are often perceived as, by their very nature, being stressful. Any approach that may increase work satisfaction is of benefit to both the individual and the organisation.

It is important within any discussion of the advantages of inter-professional teamwork to acknowledge that it may possibly not benefit the patient group. Webb and Hobdell (1980, p. 98) suggest that British social work may have misdirected its energies in the 'search for the holy grail of inter-professional collaboration' instead of increasing specialist skills which they suggest clients needed. This is perhaps a consideration for the development of team working within forensic mental health. The drive to build teams which has resulted from the Inquiries of the past (Blom-Cooper *et al.*, 1995; Suffolk Health Authority, 1996) may be re-directing energy away from developing specialist skills. It would certainly be a mistake to believe that teamwork and improved patient care are synonymous (Webb and Hobdell, 1980). Within forensic mental health it may be that some of the functions of teamwork, such as effective communication and setting of common objectives, are of value in themselves.

The issue of leadership within teams often creates tension between team members and is potentially divisive. The need for many patients to have a Responsible Medical Officer within forensic mental health settings provides inter-professional teams with a member who is, to some extent, put in the position of leader by others external to the service. It may be important, however, to separate the issues of accountability and leadership.

Within forensic psychiatry it can be argued that inter-professional team working is a necessity rather than a luxury since the dual role of providing care and ensuring the safety of others could not be provided by one individual or an individual discipline (Shepherd, 1995). Shepherd concludes that the problems faced by forensic mental health teams are formidable and identifies a number of management issues which are specific to the care of the mentally disordered offender. These include the ability for team members to share responsibility outside of the statutory duties which some professionals have and carry team responsibility for the 'transmission of information and performance of certain actions' (Shepherd, 1995, p. 119).

Parry-Jones (1986), in a description of team working within adolescent psychiatry, suggests the same when writing 'no single group, service or agency has the capacity to manage all aspects of all cases' (1986, p. 193). This sentiment translates well to the field of forensic mental health where individual cases are often long term and complex, involving elements of health, social care and the criminal justice system. The development of a team may initially require the fostering of mutual trust between group members in order that they can operate effectively together (Engel, 1994). A range of issues may face the team, which may become sources of conflict. These may be identified as being goal-related, role-related, procedural, problem solving or inter-professional matters. While this might lead to the assumption that inter-professional teams are solely about avoiding controversy a more useful view may be that they are in reality about the development of positive collaboration.

In summary, current health care practice dictates that clinicians should work in health care teams. Government directives make inter-agency working essential however little training clinicians might have in making them work effectively. The skills that are needed are not necessarily intuitive and are of most benefit if developed in the early stages of a clinician's professional development.

Communication and collaboration

Communication may be considered the single most important component of team working and therefore of inter-professional working itself. In a number of inquiries relating to homicides committed by patients within the mental health system poor communication has been identified as a crucial mediating factor in the events described (Ritchie Report, 1994; Blom-Cooper *et al.*, 1995; Suffolk Health Authority, 1996). The issue of ensuring an efficient through-flow of information between the patient, carers and other involved agencies is one that is crucial to safe care. 'Communication' includes both verbal and written and formal and informal methods of the transfer of information.

Some of the variables in teams include the method and degree of communication between members. Collaboration as such may be defined in five stages (Armitage, 1983). These are:

- Isolation
- Encounter
- Communication
- Partial collaboration
- Full collaboration

These stages in effect describe collaboration as a range from those teams where two professionals remain isolated from one another to those where all team members are involved and communicate widely and effectively. However, communication that aids rather than hinders collaboration may be restricted by the lack of common language which can be shared by all team members. Pietroni (1992) categorises team languages as being from one of many different philosophical bases. It may be impractical to expect each professional to fully understand the language of the others. It may be that the use of reflective practice within teams should be engaged in order that the different languages used are integrated with one another.

As with team working in general, the issues of both communication and collaboration are such that they are not necessarily intuitive. They are skills that need to be learned in the same way as other professional techniques. It is important that both individual clinicians and the wider organisation to which they belong acknowledge this as a responsibility that they hold jointly and ensure that there is provision for such skills to be developed.

References

Barr, H. and Waterton, S. (1994) Inter-Professional Education in Health and Social Care in the United Kingdom. CAIPE (The UK Centre for the Advancement of Interprofessional Education). Unpublished.

Blom-Cooper, L. Hally, H. and Murphy, E. (1995) *The Falling Shadow.* Duckworth, London.

Engel, C. (1994) A functional anatomy of teamwork. In A. Leathard (ed.), *Going Inter-Professional: Working Together for Health and Welfare.* Routledge, London.

Friel, C. and Chaloner, C. (1996) The developing role of the forensic community nurse. *Nursing Times*, 29, pp. 33–5.

Kane, R. (1980) Multidisciplinary teamwork in the United States: trends, issues and implications for the social worker. In S. Lonsdsale *et al.* (eds) *Teamwork in Personal Social Services and Healthcare.* Croom Helm, London.

McGrath, M. (1991) *Multidisciplinary Teamwork.* Avebury Press, Aldershot.

Parry-Jones, W. (1986) Multidisciplinary teamwork; help or hindrance? In D. Steinberg (ed.), *The Adolescent Unit – Work and Teamwork in Adolescent Psychiatry.* Chichester, Wiley

Pietroni, P. (1992) Towards reflective practice – the languages of health and social care. *Journal of Inter-professional Care*, 1, pp. 7–16.

Rawson, D. (1994) Models of inter-professional work: likely theories and possibilities. In A. Leathard (ed.), *Going Inter-professional – Working Together for Health and Welfare.* Routledge, London.

Ritchie, J.H. (Chairman), Dick, D. and Lingham, R. (1994) The Report of the Inquiry into the Care and Treatment of Christopher Clunis. HMSO, London.

Shepherd, G (1995) Care and control in the community. In J. Crichton (ed.), *Psychiatric Patient Violence: Risk and Response.* Duckworth, London.

Suffolk Health Authority (1996) The Case of Jason Mitchells: Report of the Panel of Inquiry. Duckworth, London.

Webb, A. and Hobdell, M. (1980) Co-ordination and teamwork in the health and personal social services. In S. Lonsdale *et al.* (eds), *Teamwork in Personal Social Services and Healthcare.* Croom Helm, London.

World Health Organisation (1984) The role of WHO participating centres in continuing education, specialty training and educational research. WHO: Copenhagen.

3.4 Vocational rehabilitation

Rebecca Hills

Introduction

The value of occupation to us as human beings is well documented in terms of the role it plays in helping us to maintain well-being and health. The word occupation is frequently used to mean 'work', as many occupational therapists know to their cost. In its true sense occupation refers to 'the active process of living' (Townsend, 1997, p. 18). The belief that occupation is of value in achieving and maintaining the well-being of people underpins the view that people who have mental health problems should be provided with a means to develop a pattern of regular activity and supported in maintaining this while living in the community.

Vocation rehabilitation is a term that is used to describe the preparation of individuals to return to or start work in some capacity. The value of work to an individual is immense. It allows the individual to establish a role for themselves, maintains economic security, provides social contact and in most cases structures a routine. Work promotes self-esteem, self-efficacy and reduces symptoms of mental illness (Blankertz and Robinson, 1996, p. 1216). It results in a sense of achievement and is valued by society, indeed, it was Galen (AD 172) who said that, 'employment is nature's best physician and is essential to human happiness' (quoted in Strauss, 1968, p. 663). People who are hospitalised with mental illness face a whole range of potential difficulties in their efforts to return to some form of work or employment. Those with serious mental illnesses have frequently spent prolonged periods of time in hospital, often resulting in institutionalisation. They may never have developed a work identity (Lloyd, 1995) or the early onset of their illness may have pre-empted the development of work skills (Durham, 1997). For many the financial gains are limited by their dependence on state support and they therefore lack the motivation to develop work skills.

The mentally disordered offender faces the dual difficulties of the issues related to their illness and hospitalisation and their offending history. This produces a whole range of obstacles. The individual has no recent work history, no references, a criminal record and often no developed work skills.

The world that we work in continues constantly to change: flexible working and casual working, home based working and tele-working are all developing as employers search for the most economic methods of production (Steward, 1997). These may have positive or negative effects on the potential employment of forensic psychiatric patients but neither can be ignored. This is the social context in which the rehabilitation of these individuals is set.

This section will consider the value of providing a vocational rehabilitation programme to forensic psychiatric patients and offer some suggestions as to the ways in which this may be carried out.

How useful is a vocational rehabilitation programme to mentally disordered offenders?

It is important to consider the relevance of work in the form of mainstream 'paid employment' for people who have serious mental illnesses. The majority of them do not work and 'employment rates of 8–13% are generally cited' (Blankertz and Robinson, 1996). It would seem likely that the figure for mentally disordered offenders would be even lower due to the added difficulty of their previous involvement in the criminal justice process.

However, vocational rehabilitation programmes continue to be provided by mental health professionals throughout the world despite this apparent lack of success.

O'Flynn and Ingamells (1997) suggest that this may be due to the changing trends of vocational rehabilitation leading to the use of specific models which may be effective for some people in specific situations even though it is impossible to identify the model which will be effective for a specific individual. This 'scatter-gun' approach may not achieve the required aim for mentally disordered offenders who have to contend with problems of discrimination and stigma on two counts. The issue of the provision and use of the appropriate model for both the person and the social context in which they will exist means that a variety of models should be available which provide a programme that is relevant to employment in the local area (O'Flynn and Ingamells, 1997).

The value of vocational rehabilitation may be far wider than simply the preparation of an individual for work they may, or from the statistical evidence may not, obtain on discharge from hospital. Individuals who are treated within secure environments, as many forensic mental health patients are at some point during their contact with health services, may experience occupational deprivation. This is a state in which the individual is unable to seek or maintain work due to the range of health and sociological problems which they face (Whiteford, 1997). The development of a vocational rehabilitation programme that is accessible to all may enable this deprivation to be addressed to some degree. The rehabilitation package can also address realistic development of 'core skills' (e.g. literacy, problem solving and interactive skills) (Garner, 1995).

Vocational rehabilitation provides an opportunity for the individual to practise a work role and the associated components within a safe and supported environment. It presents the individual with challenges and experiences that may not be achieved within other therapeutic activities and it establishes routines that are accepted by society.

Vocational rehabilitation in practice

The most essential factor in the provision of vocational rehabilitation programmes is the development of a strong inter-professional and inter-agency framework within which to operate. Work training in both the community, and in some cases in-patient settings, is carried out by well-established and effective independent training agencies. A number of mental health charities (e.g. MIND and NSF) deliver work training in the community, as do some organisations working specifically with offenders (e.g. NACRO). In most local areas there are a range of these organisations providing vocational opportunities, particularly National Vocational Qualifications in a range of skills and trades. Many also offer support in further development of core skills.

Within in-patient settings vocational rehabilitation programmes are more frequently provided by clinicians, often occupational therapy staff, but also nurses in some establishments. Programmes vary from the industrial therapy type scheme to individualised, specific work projects within secure units that provide opportunities for skills development to all patients without the need for external leave.

Pre-vocational programmes have also been established within some secure environments. These may be formalised to the delivery of nationally recognised programmes such as the STEP initiative for the development of programmes to meet the individual need (Garner, 1995). These may also be incorporated into day programmes and group programmes such as 'community living skills'. Alongside the need for mental health staff to work with the voluntary sector, social services and probation to ensure individual needs are addressed within the community, clinical staff within secure environments must work inter-professionally to address these issues. Occupational therapists, nurses, social workers, psychiatrists and psychologists may all have a role to play in the provision of these services and it is only with effective joint planning and working that these developments can be achieved.

References

Blankertz, L. and Robinson, S. (1996) Adding a vocational focus to mental health rehabilitation. *Psychiatric Services*, 11, pp. 1216–22.

Durham, T. (1997) Work-related activity for people with long-term schizophrenia: a review of the literature. *British Journal of Occupational Therapy*, 6, pp. 248–52.

Garner, R. (1995) Pre-vocational training within a secure environment. *British Journal of Occupational Therapy*, 1, pp. 2-6.

Lloyd, C. (1988) A vocational rehabilitation programme in forensic psychiatry. *British Journal of Occupational Therapy*, 4, p. 3.

Lloyd, C. (1995) *Forensic Psychiatry for Health Professionals*. Chapman and Hall, London.

O'Flynn, D. and Ingamells, H. (1997) *Working Together – The Network in Lewisham. A Life in the Day*. Pavillion Publishing.

Steward, B. (1997) Employment in the next millenium. The impact of changes in work on health and rehabilitation. *British Journal of Occupational Therapy*, 6, pp. 268–71.

Strauss, M.B. (1968) *Familiar Medical Quotations*. Little Brown, Boston.

Whiteford, G. (1997) Occupational deprivation and incarceration. *Journal of Occupational Science – Australia*, 4, p. 3.

3.5 A psychoeducation model for schizophrenia

Stuart Wix

Psychoeducation models and psychosocial intervention strategies in schizophrenia have gained prominence in recent years (David, 1990; Eckman *et al.*, 1990; Birchwood, 1992). Roback and Abramowitz (1979) have already demonstrated that patients who possess a degree of insight are better adjusted behaviourally during their stay in hospital, more accepting of treatment and generally tend to have a more favourable prognosis.

Patients with schizophrenia, and paranoid schizophrenia in particular, constitute the largest group in medium and high security psychiatric hospitals in the United Kingdom (Taylor, 1982; Higgins, 1998). However,

Lindquist and Allebeck (1990) have shown that people with schizophrenia have a similar rate of offending in general as the rest of the population, but are more likely to commit violent crime. Therapeutic activity in forensic psychiatry settings for schizophrenia sufferers is commonly undertaken by the individual clinicians, by a psychiatrist, psychologist or psychiatric nurse. This usually takes the form of assessment, diagnosis, treatment and rehabilitation. Patients with a diagnosis of schizophrenia who gain and develop a degree of insight, tend to achieve this in an ad hoc fashion, through their relationship with various mental health professionals, or as a result of medication or personal endeavour by seeking out help and information for themselves. There is an overall lack of understanding of the illness and its treatment by patients with this diagnosis. Individuals with a diagnosis of schizophrenia are often viewed as poor responders to 'talking therapies'. Andrews and Teeson (1994) have argued recently that medical, nursing and mental health staff trained in psychiatric hospitals view schizophrenia, erroneously, as a chronic deteriorating disease, where physical treatments are considered to be the most useful and in some cases only form of therapy, and that psychosocial interventions are commonly overlooked. They argue further that such a widely held view should not prevail as there are alternative treatment methods available.

Birchwood *et al.* (1989) pioneered 'Early Signs' work in All Saints Hospital in Birmingham. They advocated a cognitive approach to symptom management with an emphasis on acceptance and mastery of the illness. This approach used four psychosocial interventions: individual cognitive therapy, group cognitive therapy, family education and a meaningful activity programme designed to reduce negative symptoms and improve self-esteem.

One possible psychological intervention for schizophrenia in a medium secure setting is a psychoeducation model. The overall aim of a six-week programme of meetings is to empower the individual by increasing understanding of the illness, and provide an opportunity to exercise a greater degree of control and self-determination through the early recognition of signs and symptoms that would indicate relapse. Such a psychoeducation programme may be facilitated by most mental health workers, including psychiatric nurses, psychologists and psychiatrists. (See Box 3.2.)

Educational model

It is desirable that a psychoeducation programme be facilitated using a multi-method approach that is both educational and client-centred. Ewles and Simnett (1985) described the aim as being to give knowledge and ensure understanding of health issues, based on the notion that this will enable well-informed decisions to be made in future. The passage of information about the nature of 'schizophrenia', in this instance, will at least ensure that patients have a better understanding of the meaning of many of the symptoms experienced, and why specific treatments might be prescribed. With a client-centred approach, information is presented in a value-free way and individuals are helped to explore their attitudes to the illness, and to

---

Box 3.2 Schizophrenia psychoeducation programme

Aims and objectives

1 To employ suitable selection and assessment criteria which will ensure that those patients exposed to the programme will gain most benefit.

2 To introduce group members to facts regarding schizophrenia and dispel common myths.

3 To enhance the individual's level of insight into the illness of schizophrenia through discussions of causes, symptoms, the effects on behaviour, recognition of early signs and treatment.

4 To provide a forum where individuals can discuss issues surrounding the concept of 'illness' and schizophrenia in particular, in a supportive environment.

5 To achieve a level of understanding such that the possession of insight will affect future coping strategies (Kenworthy and Nicklin, 1989).

---

make their own decisions about their mental well-being. Any such programme should aim to enhance knowledge and understanding, and enable clients to discuss mental health related issues openly. The therapist adopts the role of facilitator. This ensures that discussion can occur within the group, enhances individual members' abilities to interact and improve learning outcomes. Through this educational model, material facts are given to the client to provide a knowledge base from which discussion can take place, to allow for movement to a position of empowerment and enhanced understanding toward the end of the programme.

Client selection and assessment

In establishing a small group of suitable patients who can increase their degree of insight through a psychoeducation approach, the selection process is of vital importance. Individuals who would be most likely to benefit from a psychoeducation model may already possess a degree of insight and be receiving psychotropic medication. There may be some value in having a mixture of individuals, with some in the more acute phase of the illness, with others whose symptoms are in remission.

A schedule such as the Insight Assessment Scale (Birchwood *et al.*, 1989) is a useful tool to establish an individual's awareness of their illness, need for treatment and attribution of symptoms. Although not entirely exhaustive, this provides a useful foundation in order to establish a baseline level of insight. There are other assessment tools available, including that of David (1990), but the Insight Scale is less cumbersome than most. Individuals referred for inclusion in a programme may also be screened for signs of low mood by using the Beck Depression Inventory (BDI), which is helpful in this context in identifying such factors as low self-esteem, which may hinder an individual's progress in the group of this nature (Beck, 1978).

Group content

In essence, a psychoeducation group that promotes awareness of schizophrenia, focuses upon indicators of relapse 'prodromal signs and symptoms', recognition of personal stress factors, and treatments and coping strategies.

The emphasis of the six-week package is on cooperative working to help individuals with schizophrenia develop skills and understanding that will enable them to return to the community. The first three sessions may include discussion of group members' beliefs about schizophrenia. These are then evaluated against a presentation of commonly held myths and facts about the illness. In subsequent groups the therapists present more detailed information regarding positive and negative symptoms of schizophrenia, which is reinforced with the group being shown a section of film outlining other sufferers' experience of their illness. The remaining three sessions include one that focuses on treatment and medication issues, one that examines possible self-help strategies, one that could be employed when prodromal signs are present, and one used for review and an examination of all the information given. This final meeting also allows for an evaluation of group members' understanding and experiences. (See Box 3.3.)

Box 3.3 The six-week programme

WEEK 1

 Ice-breaker (warm-up exercise)
 What is schizophrenia?

WEEK 2

 What are the features of the illness?
 Positive symptoms
 Negative symptoms

WEEK 3

 What causes schizophrenia?
 ?Inherited –
 'Street drugs'
 Video material – sufferer's perspective
 Discussion

WEEK 4

 Treatment and medication

WEEK 5

 Evaluation and pathway to help and support when living in the community:
 GP
 CPN, SW
 Psychiatry
 MIND

WEEK 6

 Video material – recap of programme content – group evaluation

---

Therapeutic strategy

Groups are often tailored to meet the differing and changing needs of individual members. This is often achieved by regularly eliciting information from group members about their levels of insight and understanding of relevant information. It is also important that the therapist adopts a non-confrontational approach to each session with material carefully tailored to the needs of the group members. Therapists in this context should also actively avoid focusing a session on individuals, particularly in relation to issues around the index offence and other personal case details. The therapist's role is to act as an educator, in the first instance, and to facilitate discussion within the group when issues are raised.

Experience has shown that a psychoeducational group of this nature is best facilitated by at least two professionals. Therapists take it in turns to lead a session, whilst the other takes notes from observations of each group member's level of participation, comments made and general conduct throughout the programme. This is an important aspect of running a group successfully as it provides the opportunity to feed back directly to clinical teams any concerns that may have arisen, and to evaluate an individual's progress, making any appropriate recommendations for future care and treatment once the programme has been completed.

The presence of two therapists enhances discussion between group members. There are occasions when discussions may become quite 'heated', particularly when an individual is challenging information that might for the first time undermine and weaken previously held notions, whether based on a delusional system or not. Two therapists can reinforce information given at the same time as well as gently questioning preconceived beliefs. This approach requires experience, skill and practice to be effective.

Evaluation

The evaluation process of the group and individual participants is as important as the selection of clients for inclusion in the programme. It is usually two-fold; first, that of the group participants where an immediate impression is attained, through verbal feedback establishing which elements of the sessions were useful and those that were not. This may lead to structural adjustments to individual sessions for future groups. The second element is to re-employ Birchwood's Insight Scale in order to assess whether a shift has occurred in the individual's overall level of understanding. The results of the follow-up assessment are incorporated into the body of a report for each patient, which outlines session by session any progress made. The report itself may be discussed with the patient, where appropriate, and that discussion may, in itself, be a positive therapeutic intervention.

References

Andrews, G. and Teeson, M. (1994) Smart treatments versus dumb treatment: services for mental disorders. *Current Opinion in Psychiatry*, 6, pp. 181–5.

Beck, A.T. (1978) *Beck Depression Inventory.* The Psychological Corporation, San Antonio, TX.

Birchwood, M. (1992) Practice review. Early intervention in schizophrenia: theoretical background and clinical strategies. *British Journal of Clinical Psychology,* 31, 257–78.

Birchwood, M., Smith, J., Macmillan, F. *et al.* (1989) Predicting relapse in schizophrenia: the development and implementation of an early signs monitoring system using patients and families and observers. *Psychological Medicine,* 19, pp. 649–56.

David, A.S. (1990) Insight and psychosis. *British Journal of Psychiatry,* 156, pp. 798–808.

Eckman, T.A., Lierberman, R.P., Phipps, C. and Blair, K. (1990) Teaching medication management skills to schizophrenic patients. *Journal of Clinical Psycho-Pharmacology,* 10, pp. 33–8.

Ewles, L. Simnett, I. (1985) *Promoting Health, A Practical Guide to Health Education.* John Wiley, Chichester.

Higgins, J. (1998) Crime and mental disorder. In D. Chiswick and R Cope (eds), *Seminars in Practical Forensic Psychiatry.* Gaskell, Redwood Press, London

Kenworthy, N. and Nicklin, P. (1989) *Teaching and Assessing Nursing Practice: An Experiential Approach.* Scutari Press.

Lindquist, P. and Allebeck, P. (1990) Schizophrenia and crime; a longitudinal follow-up of 644 schizophrenics in Stockholm. *British Journal of Psychiatry,* 157, pp. 345–50.

Roback, H.B.and Abramowitz, S.L. (1979) Insight and hospital adjustment. *Canadian Journal of Psychiatry,* 139, pp. 233–6.

Taylor, P.J. (1982) Schizophrenia and violence. In J. Gunn and D.P. Farrington (eds), *Abnormal Offenders: Delinquency and the Criminal Justice System.* John Wiley, Chichester.

3.6 Therapeutic dilemmas in forensic practice

Martin Humphreys and Norman McClelland

The nature of secure care is such that it may compromise personal freedom and civil liberties, restrict movement and place limits on a wide range of activities of daily living. This situation is, in some part at least, unique to forensic mental health practice. Forensic mental health nursing literature over the years has strongly suggested that nurses, and many other professionals, find difficulty in reconciling distinct concepts such as security and therapy, personal autonomy and the right to treatment, and the maintenance of professional boundaries within a therapeutic relationship (Burrows, 1993; Peternelj-Taylor 1998).

Issues related to what might be considered therapeutic dilemmas in forensic mental health practice range across professional boundaries, clinical settings, diagnostic groups, and patient legal categories. Difficulties of this sort may arise at any stage of a patient's contact with services, at any point in a clinician's working life, and at any time in a therapeutic relationship. Such a situation may frequently involve others, including carers, immediate family, and in some cases statutory and voluntary agencies. The impact of such therapeutic dilemmas clearly is evident, and is of increasing importance to clinicians and carers as well as users of mental health services generally and forensic services in particular (Chaloner and Kinsella, 1999; Chaloner, 2000; Evans *et al.*, 2000).

There are a number of commonly encountered situations with which the reader may be familiar in clinical practice, all of which typify and reflect the way in which the therapeutic relationship in forensic work can be compromised. These include the use of illicit substances within secure environments and beyond, dealing with hostility and physical violence, the maintenance of appropriate professional boundaries, therapeutic relationships, the difficulty of promoting innovative and creative practice in restricted environments, dealing with offender patients, as well as treatment and management of severe mental disorder in the face of issues such as terminal illness.

In the latter case a diagnosis of terminal illness gives rise to a wide variety of difficulties. There will obviously be a change in focus with regard to the overall care of an individual so diagnosed, with an overriding concern to maintain the least restrictive form of management in every sphere. Such a situation may provoke division within a multidisciplinary team, and will require a change of attitude in the team decision making process. Concerns will arise over the need to balance the requirements of individual patients, their family, and friends and the requirement to maintain public safety and observe legal constraints that may be placed upon the patient. The multidisciplinary team must manage what is essentially a grieving process for the family and carers within a secure setting. They must provide periods of privacy and the maintenance of dignity for all concerned. There may be difficulties too for other agencies who play a key part in the process such as Macmillan nurses, grief counsellors and/or befriending agencies. An associated problem is the provision of the necessary high-quality physical treatment for a dying patient in a secure environment. The core skills of the forensic mental health nurse, whilst being appropriate to a holistic approach, may not be sufficient for the specialist nature of physical care required in such a situation. Such dilemmas are made worse by the necessity to address formal risk assessment in terms of issues such as graduated leave, balancing the wish to afford the individual more liberty, perhaps in the face of worsening psychological distress and physical ill health, which may become manifest in more severe psychiatric symptoms.

There is a growing literature associated with the concern over the difficulties associated with inappropriate relationships between health care professionals in general and their patients. This is an area of particular concern in forensic mental health practice, given the intensity of the environment and the therapeutic relationship. Compromise would appear to be the key concept associated with this therapeutic dilemma, the compromise that such an inappropriate relationship can bring to patient care and to multidisciplinary team functioning, as well as both personal and professional standards (UKCC Code of Professional Conduct, 1998). This will lead to damage to the patient in terms of any potential partnership being unequal. The scope for breach of confidentiality is vastly increased in such a relationship, and has a significant effect not only on those involved in the relationship but others who know and work with either the professional concerned or the patient. The effects on others may be equally harmful with damage to other relationships in which either party might be involved, as well as being catastrophic in terms of career development and continuing risk assessment. Within a secure environment other patients who are alerted to such a relationship may be unsettled, feel threatened or compromised themselves, or be unduly concerned about the impact it might have on themselves. Colleagues may perceive a professional as having a lack of self-control and a reduced self-awareness as a consequence of becoming involved in such a relationship. Many professionals believe such a relationship compromises the degree of responsibility that a professional is able to maintain in other spheres of their work. This perceived lack of professional responsibility may lead to others questioning areas such as accurate and honest recording of signs and symptoms of illness and behaviour. The managerial responsibility in terms of how to confront an individual involved in such a relationship, either professional or patient, is an extremely difficult one. Bound up in this necessary confrontation is the manager's acknowledgement of what may be a normal expression of sexuality for a patient, coupled with the recognition of the circumstances the professional finds themselves in. The manager must be aware that the relationship may be operating on a number of different levels. The nature of secure environments is such that the residents tend to be predominantly male, referral sources range from prison settings to special hospitals and from local services to the community. Some male patients may have had little or no contact with women for some considerable time. The small number of females resident in medium secure settings may have also come from single sex environments. The potential for compromised relationships between female patients and male professionals is exacerbated by the common experience of this former group of previous abusive relationships (Peters, 1988; Stein *et al.*, 1988). Both male and female patients in secure environments are likely to have under-developed social and interpersonal skills, leading to the potential for over-dependence.

References

Burrows, S. (1993) The role of the forensic nurse. Facilitating the health management of the mentally abnormal offender. *Senior Nurse*, 13 (5), pp. 20–5.

Chaloner, C. (2000) Ethics and morality. In C. Chaloner and M. Coffey (eds), *Forensic Mental Health Nursing: Current Approaches*. Blackwell, Oxford, pp. 269–87.

UKCC (1998) Code of Professional Conduct. UKCC, London.

Chaloner, C. and Kinsella, C.(1999) The attitudes of forensic mental health nurses. In P. Tarbuck, B. Topping Morris and P. Burnard (eds), *Forensic Mental Health Nursing: Strategy and Implementation*. Whurr, London, pp. 162–70.

Evans, N. and Clarke, J. (2000) Addressing issues of sexuality. In C. Chaloner and M. Coffey (eds), *Forensic Mental Health Nursing: Current Approaches*. Blackwell, Oxford, pp. 252–69.

Peters, S.D. (1988) Child sexual abuse and later psychological problems. In Gayle Elizabeth Wyatt and Gloria Johnson-Powell (eds), *Lasting Effects of Child Sexual Abuse*. Sage, Newbury Park, Califonia, pp. 101–99.

Peternelj-Taylor, C.A. (1998) Forbidden love: sexual exploitation in the forensic mileu. *Journal of Psychosocial Nursing and Mental Health Services*, 36 (6), pp. 17–23.

Stein, J.A., Golding, J.M., Siegel, M., Burnham, A. and Sorenson, S.B. (1988) Long-term psychological sequelae of child sexual abuse: the Los Angeles epidemiological catchment area study. In Gayle Elizabeth Wyatt and Gloria Johnson-Powell (eds), *Lasting Effects of Child Sexual Abuse*. Sage, Newbury Park, Califonia, pp. 135–54.

4 Dealing with hostility

Mark West and Dave Abolins

Introduction

> Violent behaviour is a concern to both patients and staff in health care settings. Anxiety escalates, adrenaline flows and the human responses of fright, flight, and fight are often manifested; the therapeutic environment is suddenly challenged, loses stability and is temporarily thrown off balance. (Boettcher, 1983)

Violence and aggression within care settings have featured as part of everyday life for many health care workers and can be cited as common reasons for staff absenteeism. Traditional strategies for addressing the issue of aggression at work have included denial, over-reaction, or the use of large numbers of staff to manage incidents. The aftermath of aggressive incidents frequently involves the use of as-required medication, seclusion and psychological and/or physical trauma to staff and patients alike. Over the years the issues associated with violence and aggression in the workplace have attracted increased attention from health care workers. A large-scale survey of nurses' experience of violence at work led to a campaign to 'Stamp Out Violence' and reduce the incidence of violence experienced by nurses at work (*Nursing Times*, 1998). Concern for nurses' safety at work is further evidenced by the 'zero tolerance' campaign which aims to improve the situation (Department of Health, 1999).

Exposure to aggressive and violent behaviour at work appears to have significantly increased for nurses over the past twenty years. In the four-year period between 1979 and 1983, Hodgkinson *et al.* (1984) observed that the risks of assault to staff at one psychiatric hospital had doubled. It is suggested that there is a trend of increasing violence within society that is being reflected in health care settings where episodes of assault continue to increase (Blair and New, 1991).

However, it is difficult to establish clearly whether or not psychiatric inpatient violence is increasing because hospital staff frequently fail to report violent incidents (Rosenthal *et al.*, 1992). Inaccurate reporting of incidents is revealed by a survey of ambulance workers which suggested that the routine occurrence of verbal abuse has led to a failure to report it (*Journal of Occupational Health, Safety and Environment*, 1998, p. 14). Furthermore, a higher reported incidence of violence might reflect methodological differences in research, increased staff awareness, more rigorous reporting procedures, differences in staff perception and attitudes, and differing definitions of violence, rather than an actual increase in violent behaviours (Shah, 1993; Walker and Seifert, 1994). It has been suggested that society is not necessarily more violent, instead, we perceive that it is (Carlisle, 1995). In contrast though, Sullivan (1998) reports that actual physical violence is increasing within acute psychiatric units. The fact that psychiatric inpatient violence is common should not be surprising according to Crichton (1996), who suggests that many psychiatric patients are admitted to hospital following violent acts, and that 'dangerousness' remains a hospital admission criterion. However, it should be noted that the risks of being assaulted are not unique to psychiatric nurses. Poster and Ryan (1993) acknowledge that whilst much of the published literature relates to psychiatric settings, it is clear that assaults can occur in a variety of health care settings, including within patients' own homes.

Generally, the growing concern of health care workers is confirmed by the 1996 British Crime Survey (Home Office Research and Statistics Directorate, 1996), which reports that they are more likely to experience violence as a consequence of their work than the general population. In addition, Ryan and Poster (1993) report that nurses from a range of clinical settings appear to feel unsafe at work. Endorsing these observations, a Royal College of Nursing (RCN) survey revealed that most nurses feel more vulnerable in the hospitals in which they work than on the streets (*Journal of Occupational Health, Safety and Environment,* 1998). From the available evidence, the RCN (1998) believes that there is a problem of violence to nurses and that the overall situation has worsened. Supporting this belief, the Trades Union Congress (1999) reported that nurses are the most vulnerable group to physical attack at work. It may appear that nursing is becoming a more dangerous and less attractive occupation. Interestingly, the apparent shortage of qualified nurses, coupled with the growing risk of violence may further increase that risk. This would appear to support the observations of James *et al.* (1990), who note an association, albeit not statistically significant, between reduced permanent nursing staff and an increase in the number of reported violent incidents. This places nurses in a difficult position and may ultimately compromise the overall desire, duty, and ability of nurses to care for patients.

Clearly, the appropriate management of potential or actual aggression in health care settings should be within the same ethical, professional, legal, and philosophical parameters as any other aspect of care. This chapter is therefore inextricably linked to the philosophy and practices described in other parts of this book. At all times, nurses are charged with a duty of care that is described by Lord Atkin in 1932 as:

> You must take reasonable care to avoid acts or omissions which you can reasonably foresee would be likely to injure your neighbour. (UKCC, 1996)

When dealing with patients who display aggressive behaviours, it is essential that nurses fulfil their duty of care by adopting strategies for the management of the patient's behaviour which represent acts of care rather than of control alone.

Definition

There are many and varied definitions and descriptions of what constitutes aggressive behaviour within health care environments. Terms such as 'challenging behaviour', 'recalcitrant patients', or 'difficult patients' are not adequate to accurately describe and identify the exact nature of an individual patient's nursing care needs. Here the generic term 'aggressive behaviour' will be adopted to highlight relevant issues in this chapter. This is defined as 'any behaviour exhibited by a patient, within a health care environment, which has the potential to cause psychological or physical harm to themselves or others'. This is closely allied to the Department of Health's definition of work related violence which is:

> any incident where staff are abused, threatened or assaulted in circumstances arising out of their work, involving an explicit or implicit challenge to their safety, well-being or health. (Department of Health, 1999)

Aggression and its origins

Aggressive behaviour is never manifested without reason. This assertion is well supported by a range of published work that proposes a variety of different theoretical explanations. Such theories tend to congregate around the three domains of psychological, biological, and psychosocial explanation. Mackintosh (1990) identifies that attempts to explain aggression are diverse and can often be subjectively influenced by the professional background of the person offering the description. Consequently, he claims that many of the views expressed by a variety of different people are founded in advocacy rather than evidence. There are a number of different theories of aggression that might be mutually exclusive or mutually contingent. It is not the intention here to suggest a preferred theory or theories. Instead the reader is encouraged to review for themselves the various theoretical models and relate any findings to their experience and clinical practice.

Aggression in context

It should be noted that some expression of aggression by patients might be appropriate to their perception of the situation. Whilst the expression of aggression is not necessarily welcomed by patients and staff, not all aggressive behaviours exhibited by patients within health care environments are abnormally motivated. There may be many features of such a situation that are unnatural and likely to increase levels of frustration for patients using the service. Inflexible routines and practices, limited facilities, restricted access to family, friends and staff are just a few of the many possible triggers for aggression. During times of increasing frustration and limited self-control it is possible that some patients might become angry and hostile. It is therefore important that nurses are able to develop and retain a desire and aptitude to assess and understand why a particular patient might behave in the way that they do. The Department of Health and Welsh Office

(DHWO, 1999) suggest that a patient's behaviour should always be seen in context. This advice is pivotal if the unjust and unhelpful stereotyping and labelling of patients merely as 'difficult and aggressive' is to be avoided.

Ethical principles of care

According to Tarbuck (1992a), many ethical principles, including benefi-cence (to act in the best interests) and non-maleficence (to do no harm), guide the way that care should be provided to patients. These principles remain valid even at times where there is a need to manage a patient's aggressive behaviour. Furthermore, in all circumstances, there is a requirement that any care is provided within conditions that allow and encourage a co-operative approach between patient and nurse. This collaboration is not always easy, or possible, to achieve at all times with all patients and so, beneficence and non-maleficence are major guiding factors in such situations. The right to care is universal and in this respect, other ethical principles of equity, justice and fidelity are equally important.

A challenge exists for nurses who are faced with rising levels of personal anxiety and adrenaline to remain professional and objective. Such professional composure can be difficult to achieve but is vital if the natural responses of fright, flight and fight are to be appropriately managed. If nurses are unable to gain and maintain a degree of professional composure, they are more likely to respond to episodes of aggression inappropriately. During such times, it is possible that nurses cease to act professionally and compromise themselves ethically and professionally.

Prior to an aggressive incident

There are many considerations that can be addressed to reduce the likelihood of aggression within health care settings. Efforts that are aimed at prevention rather than management of such behaviours represent safer and easier strategies for nurses to adopt and maintain. There are professional and statutory obligations that have to be met. The Health and Safety at Work etc. Act (1974), the Workplace Regulations (Health and Safety Commission [HSC], 1992a), and the Management of Health and Safety at Work Regulations (HSC, 1992b) provide legislative structures that are primarily aimed at promoting the safety and well-being of all people in the workplace. The Health and Safety at Work Act (1974) specifically places responsibility on employers and employees to act reasonably to avoid hazardous working conditions by adopting safe working practices in safe working environments. Furthermore, the Workplace Regulations (HSC, 1992a) identify aspects of the working environment that must be complied with in order to provide acceptable working conditions. The Management of Health and Safety at Work Regulations (HSC, 1992b) require that there are organisational arrangements and management systems in place which relate to health and safety. These systems should incorporate, and be based upon, risk assessment with clear procedures and appropriate training for staff to be able to deal with 'dangers' such as fires or violence at work.

Education and training to support 'fit for purpose'

Organisations aspire to be associated with quality and reputation. In an ever-changing professional environment, appropriate support, supervision and education are essential ingredients for any group of workers to be successful. This responsibility is a particularly fundamental aspect of any service where carers may be exposed to the hazards of violence and aggression.

How employers identify, select and provide training appropriate to the individual needs of their service is an issue of great concern, largely due to the way in which this type of training has evolved within the care sector. The lack of a nationally identified structure has meant that people looking to provide training for their staff are often left to make informal enquiries within their personal networks and contacts. Whilst this system of personal recommendation may serve well, it is also likely to perpetuate the continued existence of inappropriate or outdated training.

The appropriate management of potential or actual aggression presents an ongoing challenge to all aspects of 'people' services, e.g. education, health care, social services, emergency services, and prisons. For many years this challenge remained unresolved within health care services where staff were not provided with appropriate training. This resulted in the 'traditional' methods of dealing with aggressive behaviours which often involved large numbers of staff, usually male, and restraint techniques which were often carried out on an ad hoc basis (McHugh *et al.*, 1995). Rosenthal *et al.* (1992) report that General Hospital staff were not routinely trained to deal with hostile behaviours, despite providing services to patients who were delirious, demented, or psychotic. However, in recent years the need for staff training has been addressed in various forms, with the most common being the provision for teaching of 'control and restraint'.

Importantly, 'control and restraint' training has raised many debates regarding its appropriateness for use within caring services. The term 'control and restraint' (often referred to as 'C&R') is used to describe a systematic approach to physical restraint which is based upon teamwork and the application of techniques which involve the flexion or extension of body joints. Prison officers developed 'control and restraint' in the late 1970s for use within Her Majesty's Prison Service and many of the techniques originate from martial arts, with Aikido having a major influence. Consequently, within care environments this type of training presents potential conflicts regarding the level of acceptability, the level of effectiveness, and the pragmatic qualities of such physical restraint skills.

Nevertheless, following the death of a psychiatric inpatient who had been restrained, one of the recommendations of the inquiry team was to provide 'control and physical restraint' training for all nursing staff working within the hospital (DoH, 1985). Subsequently, in the absence of widespread alternative training methods, 'control and restraint' training has proliferated within the National Health Service over recent years, particularly within forensic psychiatric settings. The popularity of 'control and restraint' training has been further aided by a misplaced belief that such training is approved by the Home Office. This is not the case and the Mental Health Act Commission (1997) have stated that no courses exist which are officially endorsed by the Home Office or Department of Health.

'Control and restraint' training could be viewed as encouraging aggressive responses to aggressive behaviours, and may present significant difficulty in transferring from its prison origins to health care facilities. Many health care professionals have voiced concern regarding the use and abuse of 'control and restraint' techniques (RCN, 1992; Tarbuck, 1992a, 1992b; Topping-Morris, 1995; Royal College of Psychiatrists, 1998).

This aspect of nursing is extremely contentious and has attracted much attention, resulting in some training courses attempting to distance themselves from their origins of 'control and restraint'. However, many of them have merely disguised their origins and been content to adopt euphemistic terminology. Unfortunately, the fact that nurses are occasionally required to physically restrain patients is inescapable, so methods that are judged as 'acceptable' should be used at all times. The philosophy that underpins course curricula, and the way in which courses are taught, may impact upon patient care. Importantly, the conflicts and difficulties presented by the use of 'control and restraint' in health care environments should be addressed through developments within course content, structure, and the types of physical restraint skills taught.

A major flaw of many early courses was that whilst people were taught very effective ways of using methods of physical control and restraint, the courses failed to properly address the issues concerned with avoiding violent incidents occurring in the first place. This left gaps in the areas of prevention and de-escalation, and developments beyond the initial holding and restriction of movement were not made. Such developments are crucial if training is to reflect current ideologies and practice. The primary focus of training should be upon prevention and non-physical methods of working with aggressive clients. It is equally clear that the teaching of physical techniques to certain groups of staff might be appropriate but the UKCC (1998a) reinforce the notion that physical restraint should be used as a last resort.

Focusing upon terminology can often be seen as pedantic but it is important that any description accurately reflects practice. Euphemisms can create mental images and implied attitudes that do not necessarily represent practical reality (i.e. different terminology does not necessarily indicate different skills). Historically the term 'control and restraint' has been used to describe the training provided to nurses on how to manage aggressive patient behaviours. Unfortunately, in some instances, military-style phrases were used to communicate between the team and to the patient. Whilst this was intended to offer structure and clarity of communication in difficult situations, they might also be considered to detract from the notion of a positive human interaction. Therapeutic working with clients in crisis requires a form of interaction that aims to strengthen the relationships between clients and those who care for them. Not only did the use of military language potentially de-humanise the process but it also tended to make life for course participants more difficult because they were expected to learn new terms to replace those that came naturally. The emphasis upon communication during aggressive episodes cannot be overemphasised. It is essential that all communication is meaningful and aspires to restore and strengthen the client and carer relationship.

As attitudes matured towards the content of training courses, some trainers started to develop alternative methods to the original skills and principles that they had learned. It was clear that physical skills taught needed to be more client-focused and highly client-sensitive. In addition, it was considered to be inappropriate to teach physical skills for dealing with violence and aggression in isolation from the subjects of prevention and de-escalation. Consequently, some courses were developed that offered the teaching of physical skills alongside theoretical elements relating to care and prevention. The RCN (1992) document 'Seclusion, Control and Restraint' sets out guidelines for good practice and makes specific comment regarding the availability, content, delivery, supervision and control of 'control and restraint' courses for nursing staff.

In 1993 the English National Board for Nursing, Midwifery and Health Visiting (ENB) issued a circular that indicated that studies concerning violence and aggression should be included within all pre-registration nurse training programmes. It further described two new courses 'Coping with Violence and Aggression: Effective Prevention and Management Techniques for Practitioners' (ENB 956: Stage 1 and ENB 769: Stage 2). The ENB (1993) document included a section titled 'Specification for Control and Restraint Instructors' that described the required characteristics of trainers who should be involved in teaching physical interventions on these ENB educational programmes. At that time, the ENB did not propose to offer courses that would train the trainers and subsequently, it became apparent that many 'control and restraint instructors' did not meet the outlined specification. As a result, the University of East Anglia developed a course curriculum that captured the elements of the specification and by 1995 the ENB had validated this as a programme which would appropriately develop and prepare people to become trainers. The new course was titled 'Training the Trainers – Control and Restraint Techniques for Nurses, Midwives and Health Visitors on all parts of the Professional Register' and as a centre-generated programme, became referred to as the ENB A74.

Also in 1993, members of the RCN Forum for Nursing in a Controlled Environment publicly raised the issue of 'control and restraint' training. They voiced concern over the continued lack of standards and also the credibility of trainers providing courses for care workers. As a consequence, they liaised with the RCN Institute (RCNI) and drafted an outline curriculum for training the trainers. This curriculum document forms the basis of current programmes that enable people to become RCNI prepared trainers in the management of actual or potential aggression.

A system for identifying people who have successfully completed an approved programme is now established. This can provide accessible information to prospective or existing training providers when looking for appropriate trainers in the field of aggression management. The RCNI maintain a register of trainers and the admission and periodic re-registration criteria aim to ensure that the standards of 'best practice' identified for RCNI prepared trainers are maintained. This on-going process serves to safeguard the interests of clients, carers and their employers regarding the appropriateness and quality of RCNI prepared trainers and any services offered by them. Attitudes displayed during courses by trainers can have a dramatic impact on the notion of delivering care during a crisis and consequently, the RCNI published a Code of Professional Conduct for RCNI prepared trainers to follow (RCNI, 1997).

It is important to stress the interdependence of the theoretical and practical components of all training programmes. The RCNI recognise that a published set of minimum standards are required in order to ensure that all courses delivered by trainers held on their records address the key non-physical aspects associated with the care and management of actual or potential aggression. They produced a set of minimum training standards (RCNI, 1997) which make comment upon course monitoring, content, group size, student ratio, duration of training, training environments, and general personal safety. The teaching of physical skills is aimed at enabling carers to work therapeutically with clients during times of crisis and, therefore, no physical restraint skills taught by RCNI prepared trainers are designed or intended to harm or hurt the client. The focus on client sensitivity cannot be overemphasised.

The future of training in this area for nurses lies in the professional preparation and maintenance of trainers in the management of actual or potential aggression. It is essential that these 'trainers' possess professional credibility and competence to be able to place the content and context of training programmes within the ethical and professional boundaries of nursing.

Proactive strategies of care

Individualised patient care is a fundamental requirement in modern health care services. Consequently, if this concept and approach is to apply to everyone, including those patients who express aggressive behaviours, it is essential that care plans incorporate strategies to prevent and manage aggressive behaviours. Comprehensive and ongoing assessments should reveal important information that can aid the compilation of appropriate and effective individualised strategies of care. In terms of avoiding aggressive behaviour, the establishment of a therapeutic environment is likely to be helpful. With this in mind, it is helpful to consider the acronym 'PUNCH' (Figure 4.1) to consider the factors that are important to a therapeutic environment.

Patient

Ongoing assessment
It is essential that the assessment process determines where a patient is most likely to benefit from being placed. Furthermore, comprehensive assessment information is likely to provide significant guidance in the identification of appropriate care strategies for patients. Stirling (1998) suggests that there is an identifiable continuum of violence that can help to identify tangible points which patients might pass through during escalation from a state of calm control to violence (Figure 4.2).

The following clinical example illustrates the violence continuum (Stirling, 1998).

Patient

Ongoing assessment

Appropriately placed
Fully informed
Actively involved in care

Unobtrusive observation

Effective

Dangerous behaviours and contraband items
Therapy and security needs balanced

Nurses

Genuine and honest

Professional and skilled
Motivated and non-judgemental
Consistent practice by unified teams

Communication

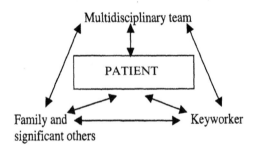

Healthy environment

Safe and comfortable

Resources and activities
Privacy, space, and time
Contact with the 'outside world'

Figure 4.1 Therapeutic environment – avoiding aggressive behaviour

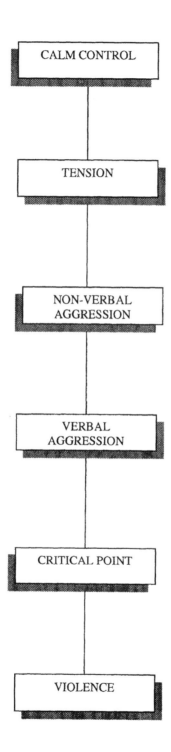

Figure 4.2 The violence continuum (Stirling, 1998)

Case study: Mr J

Mr J was admitted to the acute admission area of the clinic. Initially he presented as psychotic and expressed a range of intense delusions. At times he was difficult to manage and sometimes became violent. His violence was usually directed at other patients and staff who became incorporated into his abnormal beliefs. A relatively short period of assessment identified an observable pattern of escalating behaviour:

- **Calm control:** *Mr J did not present aggressive behaviour at all times. For lengthy periods he appeared to be in a state of relative calm and interacted freely with staff and other patients.*
- **Tension:** *There were a number of early warning signs that suggested all was not well. Mr J would remove himself from communal areas and retire to his bedroom to play loud music.*
- **Non-verbal aggression:** *After a while he would return to the communal areas and begin to pace the floor whilst looking troubled and pre-occupied. Often he would rush back to his room and slam the door shut.*
- **Verbal aggression:** *Mr J would begin to target an individual patient or member of staff and accuse them loudly of interfering with his brain. His manner would be hostile and intimidating. He would then usually disengage to leave the scene and return briefly to his bedroom.*
- **Critical moment:** *Mr J would return to the communal area to further rebuke the identified victim whilst standing inches away from them.*
- **Violence:** *If the victim said nothing or backed away, Mr J would follow them until they became confronting about his behaviour, or tried to push him away. Mr J would then engage in a short frenzied assault, using his fists to aim blows to the other person's head.*

Recognising and becoming familiar with this pattern of behaviour allowed nurses to produce proactive intervention strategies that focused upon preventing or reducing an escalation of behaviour which would result in aggression or violence.

The utilisation of the violence continuum (Stirling, 1998) might elicit observable patterns of behaviour that could be incorporated into a nursing model for assessment and care planning. In this respect, a variety of models exist to formalise and structure the assessment process. Boettcher (1983) (Figure 4.3) proposes a model for nursing the violent individual within a care environment that is based upon an analysis of nine human needs. Adopting this model might provide useful structure to the assessment of the underlying reasons for a patient's behaviour. Appropriate care strategies could then be identified, which are likely to eliminate or reduce the impact of the identified aggressive behaviour.

Appropriately placed

The appropriateness of the placement for any patient can significantly affect the ability to provide a therapeutic environment. If patients are inadequately assessed or inappropriately placed, then the patient's needs may not be properly addressed, detracting from the therapeutic potential of the placement. If an acutely ill patient is placed within an environment that is primarily geared towards rehabilitation interventions and activities, the facilities available and the focus of the staff might not adequately address the specific needs of the patient. In this situation therapeutic value is compromised for the acutely ill patient and for other patients in the same environment.

Fully informed

It is more likely that patients will retain a sense of autonomy and security, and be less likely to feel threatened and therefore hostile, in situations where they feel that they have sufficient information. In this respect it is essential that patients are engaged in discussions about their care wherever possible. There may be occasions where patients are so acutely ill that their ability to engage and understand the implications of information are limited. However, the patient's right to information remains absolute and all efforts should be made to ensure that the patient is kept as fully informed as possible in the context of their ability to understand and benefit from such information. Many patients within forensic psychiatric inpatient services are detained under the Mental Health Act 1983 (DoH, 1983) and they have rights that relate to issues such as appealing against detention and treatment. It is expected that patients are made aware of their rights on admission by being provided with the relevant information, both verbally and in writing. Not all patients are able to understand the information provided at that particular time due to their mental state. Consequently, the mandate to keep patients fully informed about their legal status, as well as other aspects of their care, should be met by ongoing review of the patient's ability to understand. Based on such reviews, further opportunities must be provided to help the patient to appreciate their rights.

Actively involved in care

Effective treatment strategies are founded upon a therapeutic alliance between patients and health care professionals. For such an alliance to form and be maintained, patients must feel that they are the focus of discussion, that they are listened to, and that they are able to contribute to, and have an investment in any treatment plan. Mental health professionals are tasked with a responsibility to keep patients involved in compiling and engaging in planned activities and treatments that are considered to be helpful. Ultimately, compliance with treatment is significantly aided by establishing agreement and a strong alliance between the patient and professional. Such a process of interaction and discussion is aimed at empowering patients who, as a result, are more likely to experience less anxiety and frustration regarding their care and treatment. Anecdotal evidence suggests that a failure to involve patients in planning their care and treatment can result in reduced compliance and/or increasing points of conflict.

Unobtrusive observation

Effective

The observation of patients might be part of specific security arrangements within a ward environment and also provides much valuable assessment information. It is important that observation is effective and that staff are fully aware of the precise purpose of observation for the general ward

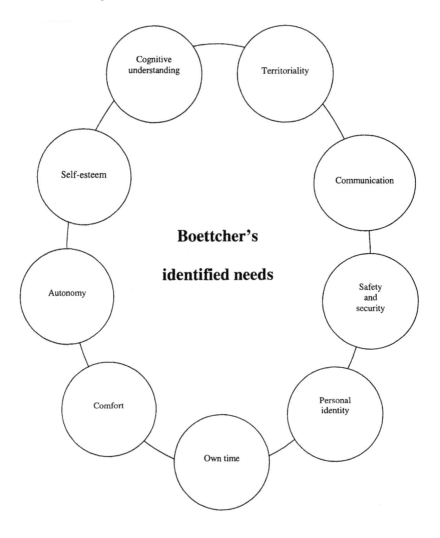

Figure 4.3 Boettcher's (1983) identified needs

population and also for specific patients. Observation is probably most effective when nurses are interacting with patients. In these situations, it is likely that the observation is less obtrusive and more discreet and a more acceptable method of observing patients than from a distance. Despite this, there might be times when it is inappropriate or difficult to interact and engage with patients. It is then important that effective observation continues to take place discreetly nevertheless. It is possible that some patients might require direct observation from a distance at times, for example if a patient becomes irritable in the company of others and chooses to isolate themselves. In this situation, it is important that the distance from the nurse to the patient is assessed to allow effective and unobtrusive observation that is appropriate for that particular patient at that particular time. Discreet methods of observation might serve to reduce the potential for conflict arising out of a sense of unnecessary intrusion for the patient.

Dangerous behaviours and contraband items

It is important that every care environment represents a safe place for all patients and staff. It is essential that staff are fully aware of the different types of behaviour that might be identified as early warning signs which precede a particular patient's aggressive behaviour. This information would ordinarily be elicited through observation, risk assessment, clinical notes, care planning and historical information sources It is important for staff to identify clearly and to understand what types of item are contraband for reasons of safety or security within any particular environment. Observation plays a significant part in the detection and avoidance of such items becoming readily available.

Therapy and security needs balanced

Reasonable steps are required which aim to establish a least restrictive environment and strategy for caring for each patient as an individual. It is possible that over-emphasis of security issues might compromise the potential to maximise treatment and therapeutic interactions. Conversely, it is possible that inadequate security provision might fail to provide a safe environment for the successful treatment and interventions, or safe accommodation for patients whose behaviour might represent a danger to themselves or others. Forensic practice is concerned with providing care in secure and safe conditions for mentally disordered offenders, or others requiring similar services. Whilst it is important to acknowledge the legal and professional requirements for safe and secure health care provision for this client group, it is equally important to establish security arrangements which are appropriate to the needs of individual patients. 'Blanket' security arrangements (that is, levels of security which are applied for all patients but are based upon the minimum required for the most dangerous patient), are likely to compromise the individual needs of some patients and conflict with the concept of individualised care. Within a medium-secure unit, therapeutic values must be balanced carefully with the need to maintain sufficient and appropriate levels of care and security. The fact that patients can expect to be treated in the least restricted environment which is appropriate to their needs is highlighted by the DoH (1997). When patients display aggressive behaviours, this places great pressure upon services to ensure that they are acting within the guidelines provided by the Code of Practice, or to be able to give sufficient justification for departing from its identified standards. It is anticipated that an individualised approach to care and security is more likely to create conditions that promote a patient's ability for autonomy. Providing patients with information about their individual observation levels fulfils the notion of keeping patients fully informed and actively involved in their care. When they have information which increases their understanding of the situation, patients are more likely to be able to take greater control of themselves in order to significantly reduce the number of potentially provoking factors within their daily living environment. Such individualised approaches are helped significantly by adopting security arrangements that are based more upon human interaction than environmental constraints alone. The Special Hospitals Service Authority (SHSA) noted that an expectation for patients to become violent resulted in custodial attitudes amongst the staff of a 'special care' unit (SHSA, 1993). It might appear that the expectation for violence created a more security-conscious environment that had the paradoxical effect of making violence more likely.

Nurses

Honest and genuine

It is expected that registered nurses provide honest information to patients, and in the event that they decide to be selective with the information, the decision must be based upon the best interests of the patient (UKCC, 1996). However, it is clear that the UKCC (1996) will not condone a registered nurse being untruthful. In this respect it is evident that a nurse who is honest and genuine with patients is more likely to be able to establish the therapeutic alliance which will ultimately be of benefit to the patient. Nursing is based upon human interaction aimed at promoting the well-being of patients. Nurses must adopt the general guiding principles of human interaction in order to establish strong relationships with patients which are founded upon mutual trust, respect and understanding. It is evident that the nurses who have made the effort to establish and invest in a relationship with the patient are more able to interact effectively with patients. A lack of honesty and genuineness from nurses towards patients is more likely to foster a lack of trust or superficial relationships that are unlikely to nurture the desired degree of co-operative working.

Professional and skilled

Registered nurses must undertake to maintain and develop their professional competence and knowledge in order to comply with their Code of Professional Conduct (UKCC, 1992). This point is further reinforced by the UKCC (1998a), who advocate evidence based practice which is derived from research activity, reflections on previous experience, knowledge, and recognised standards or protocols. The need to inter-link theory with practical experience is also identified by the ENB (1998), who consider that professional practice must be based upon education and training:

> Effective education and training are the bedrock of professional practice which aims to provide the highest standards of care for patients. (ENB, 1998)

When working in areas where patients might present aggressive behaviours, this requirement is of paramount importance. Nurses require structured opportunities to reflect and develop their personal understanding and skills in the prevention and management of aggressive patients if they are to be able to make a significant impact upon the occurrence of aggression within health care settings.

Motivated and non-judgemental

Nurses who are demonstrably motivated towards patient care are more likely to be able to forge strong professional relationships with patients.

Similarly, patients are more likely to be able to relate and communicate with nurses who do not appear to judge them. In forensic services, some patients are known to have been involved in activities which that society would identify as unacceptable (for example, assault and sexual offences). In these cases it is important that nurses are able to remain non-judgemental and objective by ensuring that the ethical principle of equity (Tarbuck, 1992a) is applied to all. It is interesting to note that Stockwell (1972) suggests that certain illnesses and symptoms are likely to make patients less attractive (for example, negative attitudes are likely to be exhibited towards conditions that involve mental disturbance). This might explain the observations of the SHSA (1993), who suggest that the sense of ever-present danger which was evident in the atmosphere of a forensic ward was a result of staff attitudes as well as the disturbed nature of the patients. This comment might appear to support the observations of Rosenham (1973/1991), who noted that hospital staff did not consider themselves or the environment to be contributory or influential to a patient's behaviour:

> Never were the staff found to assume that one of themselves or the structure of the hospital had anything to do with a patient's behaviour. (Rosenham, 1973/1991, p. 9)

Consistent practice by unified teams
It is beyond doubt that one of the strengths of the nursing profession is the diversity of personalities and experience that individual nurses can bring to the health care environment. However, this strength can also become a significant disadvantage if nurses within teams work individually rather than collaboratively. It is more likely that nurses are able to utilise their individuality to the benefit of patients if they practise within an observable framework that has been agreed and is understood by the whole team. Such working practices should be based upon structured care planning procedures that are able to readily identify the goals and strategies of care for individual patients. Significantly, appropriate contingency and pre-planning would appear to positively impact upon the eventual outcome of aggressive incidents. It is therefore important that care teams are well briefed and supported by clearly defined intervention strategies that aim to address the needs of patients and of the environment. Put simply, we plan to fail if we fail to plan.

Communication

Communication is a fundamental human need and also an essential component of assessment and care. Nurses must identify and support networks of communication that are identified as being important to the welfare and well-being of the patient. These channels would include all sources of information. The collection and appropriate sharing of information impacts directly upon care. Services should encourage communication between relevant parties within the necessary bounds of confidentiality.

Healthy environment

Safe and comfortable

The health care environment should not represent a hazardous setting and of all of the features of a therapeutic environment, safety must be considered the most important. Care should be delivered in a safe way and under safe conditions. Feeling safe is important for patients who might be vulnerable because of a presence, or lack, of familiar features. It is possible that some patients might feel threatened by the behaviour of other patients within the same environment. In situations where patients or staff feel unduly threatened, high levels of stress might increase the potential for over-cautious nursing practices, resulting in custodial attitudes which may in turn increase the risk of aggression occurring. Alternatively, it is possible that some people might be unable to control their feelings of fright, flight, or fight and become aggressive in response to any perceived threat that they experience. In any event, a sense of safety within a health care environment will help to minimise the occurrence of aggression and the consequences of any displayed aggression. Attention to the use of daylight, lighting and colour might help to make environments less harsh and stimulating, and more homely and relaxed. The work of Schauss (1985) suggests that the use of a certain colour in an environment might impact upon people's behaviour. Noise levels can also be a source of stimulation and irritation to some patients, and nurses should therefore try to ensure that excessive noise from televisions or music is avoided.

Resources and activities

Inflexible routines and a lack of resources and activities are likely to result in boredom and frustration for patients that might lead to increasing levels of stress and reduced levels of self-control. It is important that we seek to provide activities that are meaningful, beneficial and valued by patients. Hallberg *et al.* (1990) observed that vocally disruptive patients were more physically dependent upon the staff but did not receive significantly different care to their contemporaries. Furthermore, they found that patients were left to themselves for 71 per cent of the time and were consequently reduced to inactivity and solitude (Hallberg *et al.*, 1990). Patients who present aggressive tendencies should be encouraged to engage with staff to enable assessment, monitoring and therapeutic work in order to reduce the likelihood of aggressive behaviour. Appropriate activities might occur within and outside of the immediate environment and would include board games, occupational therapy, educational activities, sports games, and individual fitness programmes. Inadequate resources might restrict the availability of activities and this could become a source of frustration in itself. It is important to establish activities that are realistic within the resources available, and to negotiate and agree those activities with individual patients.

Privacy, space, and time

'Hospital wards are unnatural environments' (Royal College of Psychiatrists, 1998, p. 1a). In health care settings it is important to provide conditions that allow patients to be cared for in a least restrictive and imposing way. Patients must be afforded levels of privacy that are assessed as being safe. Giving patients access to space and the ability to be able to conduct their lives at their own pace might avoid negative perceptions of control that may increase the patient's feelings of intrusion, resentment, and aggressive response. Nurses therefore, should ensure that health care environments take account, and support the notion of these basic human needs for patients who are temporarily living in an unnatural environment.

Contact with the 'outside world'

It is entirely possible that some patients could become isolated from their local community contacts and society particularly where, as in secure settings, average length of stay may be longer than elsewhere. It is important that nurses encourage the maintenance of contacts with significant others and the patient to take an active interest in societal issues. Some patients admitted to forensic facilities may be a considerable distance from their home. In these circumstances, the importance of retaining local contacts is significantly more important for the patient. In hospital the ability to communicate with the 'outside world' can be supported by the availability of telephones and stationery. Flexible visiting hours and sufficient resources and facilities to allow visits to occur in a safe and appropriate environment are obviously also important.

During an aggressive incident

De-escalation: principles and practice

De-escalation involves many different skills and strategies and, conse-quently, is likely to be interpreted in a variety of ways. The RCN (1997) describe de-escalation as a process that defuses a patient's expressed anger or aggression in order for a calmer state to ensue. Stirling (1998) (see Figure 4.2) describes a violence continuum that suggest that people have the potential to be calm as well as a potential to be violent. His work outlines five transitional stages that punctuate the escalation from calm control into violence, and further suggests that it is important for nurses to recognise these stages in order to prevent further escalation and to promote a return to a calmer state. The importance of de-escalation strategies in dealing with aggressive behaviour cannot be understated and often their use is likely to support the concepts of 'least restrictive' and 'acceptable' practice. Furthermore, the UKCC (1998a) advocate that psychological and commu-nication de-escalation techniques should ordinarily be used to defuse confrontational and challenging behaviour.

It is important to acknowledge that the successful use of de-escalation skills to manage aggressive behaviour does not occur by chance alone. Nurses must learn, practise and refine their skills of de-escalation if they wish to increase their effectiveness in managing aggression at work. According to Stevenson (1991), a basic knowledge of de-escalation skills is required to enable nurses to use their personal resources most effectively. A nurse's ability successfully to defuse aggression relies upon a combination of positive personal attributes, knowledge of the aggressor, and insight into the subtle rules of social interaction. The use of personal attributes and interpretation of the rules governing the interaction can significantly affect the behaviour of the patient.

De-escalation most frequently occurs before a situation is allowed to escalate into actual aggression or violence. Indeed, many of the preventative strategies highlighted earlier in this chapter could themselves be considered as methods of de-escalation. The appropriate prevention and management of aggression within health care settings is complex and there is overlap between prevention and de-escalation strategies. When faced with circumstances in which a patient is demonstrating a propensity for aggressive behaviour, nurses should be concerned with identifying and adopting methods of de-escalation which are likely to be suitable in that particular situation. No single definitive method of de-escalation will address the needs of every individual event. One key theme that does seem to be generally useful is that it is usually better to avoid responding to aggression with aggression. There are times when it might be difficult to control the human reactions to threat of 'fright, flight or fight', but nurses must endeavour to avoid a response of 'fight'.

In their work, McHugh *et al.* (1995) illustrate that nurses require a range of options in order to be able to respond appropriately to situations of aggression (Figure 4.4). An important feature of this de-escalation model is the ability of the nurse to be able continually to review and evaluate the feedback from the patient in relation to the option being selected. It is possible that successful strategies have been identified within assessment procedures and care plans. However, ongoing review is also likely to allow the nurse to be flexible in selecting the most appropriate option that is based upon the patient's response in a particular situation. The de-escalation model expects that self-review will occur during the interaction, and that nurses should continually review their strategy in light of the patient's response. Consequently, it is important that nurses are prepared to alter their strategy, back away or pass the conversation on to someone else if things are going badly. The ability to be flexible and make changes as appropriate within an aggressive situation should not be viewed as failure, indeed it may reflect sensible pro-active decision making.

Communication

Clearly, it is important to establish communication at some level in order to de-escalate aggression and this process is significantly aided in situations where nurses have invested in establishing a therapeutic relationship with patients before they become aggressive. The effectiveness of verbal and non-verbal de-escalation techniques can often depend upon the pre-crisis relationship between the nurse and the patient. It is important, however, to highlight that the successful de-escalation of aggression does not necessarily entail snuffing it out completely. The unnatural features of many health care environments or patient circumstances might be sufficient to provoke aggressive behaviours within the context of a 'normal response'. In these circumstances, it is sometimes helpful to restore 'acceptable' levels of aggression which are considered to represent a low level of harm and will ultimately allow patients to take control of themselves. Interactions that encourage patients to respond naturally and manage their responses appropriately are likely to be more effective in the longer term in helping patients to integrate and live in society. Nevertheless, whether the intention is to extinguish or reduce the levels of aggression, de-escalation is not a scientific process with irrefutable evidence to suggest that certain strategies are guaranteed to work in all cases.

Communication is a process of information exchange between people. It has been suggested that communication between two people involves a 'source' and a 'receiver' (Shannon and Weaver, 1949), between which a message is transmitted. However, Myers and Myers (1985) suggest that the process is dynamic and each communicator is both a 'source' and 'receiver'. Clearly, communication is a complicated process that occurs at two levels during aggressive incidents: verbal and non-verbal. Nurses must be acutely aware of the possibilities of misinterpretation of their verbal and non-verbal interactions by patients, and of their own potential to misinterpret patients' interactions. The potential for misinterpretation is likely to be greater in circumstances where a patient is highly aroused, and/or suffering an illness. In the absence of 'guaranteed methods' of de-escalation, guiding principles for these two types of communication are offered.

Verbal communication
Consider your own tone of voice and try to speak calmly, avoiding sudden changes in level and pitch. Speak slowly and clearly, using short sentences that can be repeated with quiet assertion to increase clarity if necessary. Patients who are highly aroused might not be able to listen to, or understand, your words and may become increasingly irritable if you use long rambling sentences. If you have to give instructions, explain them clearly and concisely, in stages.

Avoid giving information or discussing topics that are likely to further provoke the situation, but do not be dishonest.

Do not attempt to dominate any verbal interaction and remember that a useful rule of thumb is to use one's two ears and one mouth in proportion to each other. Active listening is more likely to indicate your interest and concern for the patient. Demonstrate that you are listening and clarify issues by the use of paraphrasing, reflection, and summarising key points. Importantly, it is often useful to engage the patient by nodding your head and encouraging them to talk by using phrases like 'I can see that you are angry' or 'Please carry on, that's really important'. The effects of these responses can often convey the fact that this issue is important, that the patient's behaviour has been noted, and that the nurse is willing to give the patient time and help to address the difficulty.

It is often useful to describe the positive choices available to the patient and thus help to increase their feelings of empowerment and autonomy. It is noteworthy that some aggressive patients who find that they have placed themselves in a position of no return might welcome alternative options which allow them a 'face-saving' way out of the conflict situation.

Non-verbal communication
During any interaction with an aggressor it is important to consider how we can use our presence most effectively and safely. This will enable us to

establish rapport, avoid provocation and importantly, maintain our personal safety. Effective verbal interactions are more likely to occur where an aggressive patient feels able to accept the presence of the person offering the proverbial 'olive branch', even in situations where there is reluctant acceptance.

Effective verbal communication can be difficult when faced with hostility. Nurses may feel anxious and under pressure to succeed, particularly if an audience is present. Choosing the right words to say in these situations may be difficult, but perhaps how we say things is more important than the words that we use.

An angry person, particularly someone who is physically hostile and aggressive, will often require a larger area of personal body space and will be extremely wary of advances towards, or intrusions into their personal zone. Consequently, nurses should attempt to avoid approaching 'head on' as this may be viewed as provocative. If the environment allows, nurses will often be perceived as less provocative and confrontational if they are able to approach or interact with an aggressive patient from a sideways position or at a 45 degree angle. Additionally, if faced with someone who is highly aroused, nurses should be prepared to stop several feet away to make an initial assessment of the situation. A larger distance might offer a relatively higher degree of safety when compared to a smaller distance, but might also help to avoid further provocation. It is important that nurses are sufficiently close to aggressive patients to be able to establish a rapport without shouting or struggling to listen, but this should not be at the expense of safety and therefore, they should keep out of easy striking distance.

Being towered over by another person can be intimidating for some people and is likely to be provocative to a highly aroused aggressive individual. Furthermore, an imbalance of height might make partnership and rapport difficult to establish and maintain. Therefore, before beginning any dialogue nurses should attempt to position themselves at the same height as the patient.

Be mindful that an angry person who may be feeling threatened by a situation, might pay more attention to what nurses are doing than to what is being said, and could easily be intimidated by sudden movements or ill-timed gestures. Similarly, sudden movements are likely to distract from any process of verbal negotiation. Folded arms, clenched fists, pointing fingers and hands in pockets should be avoided because these behaviours can easily be interpreted by an aggressive patient as indicators of hostility, disinterest, or a lack of respect. Reassuring open-handed gestures are often better received by highly aroused people than those previously described.

The appropriate use of eye contact is vital to any attempt to defuse. Intense prolonged eye contact, particularly during any period of silence, could further provoke the aggressor and may imply an equally aggressive stance from the nurse. Some eye contact is important in order to demonstrate a desire to listen and understand, and also so that the behaviour of the aggressive patient can be observed and monitored for assessment and safety reasons. The unwritten guideline for appropriate eye contact appears to be 'make it and break it'. This is probably best achieved by alternating between direct eye contact and looking towards the shoulder or chest area of the person. Thus, when direct eye contact is not being made, nurses remain able to 'see' the patient at all times by using their peripheral vision capabilities. It should be noted that if the patient is likely to assault the nurse, the assault is most likely to occur during a break in direct eye contact.

Attempting to match the mood of the aggressor can often prove useful. It is important, however, that the nurse does not become equally physically aroused or aggressive. The nurse's response should endeavour to demonstrate increased concern and a desire to find a solution to the problem by using body language which suggests a genuine but controlled degree of arousal.

Autonomy

Within modern health care practice, respect for patient autonomy is a significant theme which is supported by the Department of Health (1995, 1997) who highlight the rights of patients to receive information and clear explanations of treatment. Respect for a patient's autonomy embraces the concepts of freedom and liberty, but is not absolute and is subject to reason (Rumbold, 1993). Clearly, autonomy does not mean that patients can do whatever they wish and this point is particularly important when considering the autonomy of those patients who are aggressive. Mental health professionals often face difficult ethical choices according to Sullivan (1998), because they are expected to provide care and also to meet the demands of society to control difficult behaviours. This point is reinforced by the Department of Health and the Welsh Office (1999), who state that staff must make a balanced judgement between promoting an individual's autonomy and fulfilling their duty to protect that person from harm.

Negotiation

Successful negotiation is more likely to occur in situations where patients are interacting with staff whom they respect and feel able to trust. The importance of establishing strong professional relationships with patients cannot be underestimated. By doing so nurses are more likely to be able to use their privileged relationship to support the process of negotiation. Negotiation can only occur in conditions of honesty and the sharing of information. Its value in an aggressive situation is likely to be based upon generating a process of mutual thought and consideration of the options available, and ultimately attempting to empower the patient so far as is possible. It is helpful to the negotiation process if is has flexibility and creative approaches but within clearly defined boundaries.

Treatment

The Patient's Charter (DoH, 1997) highlights that patients should be treated in the least restricted environment which is appropriate to their needs. The successful de-escalation of patients who are aggressive is likely to be helped by clearly demonstrating this notion to them as opposed to responses that suggest 'most restrictive' and unjust practice, for example large numbers of people standing around a patient. There are strong links between de-

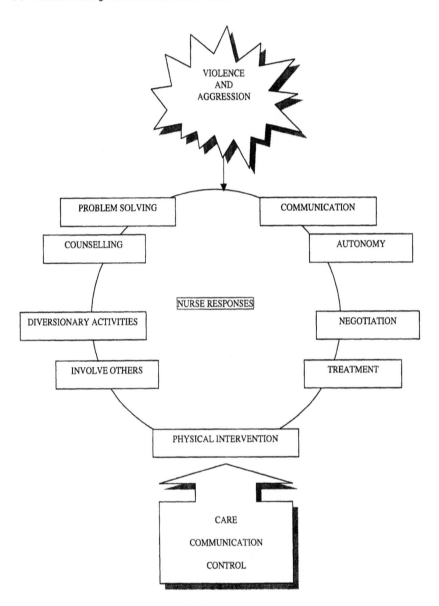

Figure 4.4 The de-escalation model (McHugh *et al.*, 1995)

escalation and care planning which is aimed at identifying the needs of patients and proposing strategies to meet those needs. Consequently, the whole notion of treatment for patients who are assessed as being likely to become aggressive, includes issues such as psychological therapies, informed consent, the Mental Health Act (DoH, 1983), and the administration of prescribed medication. Treatment plans should account for the likely occurrence of aggression in identified patients and therefore, the implementation of the plan could be considered as being part of the preventative strategy and/or the de-escalation process.

Problem solving

It is clear that wherever aggressive behaviour is exhibited, efforts to de-escalate the behaviour should incorporate strategies to address the causation or trigger factors responsible. Methods that combine calming activities with solution-focused interactions and commitment are likely to be more effective than those that do not. Nurses who interact with aggressive patients in a manner that clearly illustrates that they want to help to deal with relevant issues rather than just calm them down, are more likely to encourage patient cooperation. It is probably better for nurses to provide patients with information and guidance so that they can identify solutions for themselves rather than merely accepting solutions offered to them. Clearly, solutions cannot always be immediate and it should be noted that agreeing a plan with the patient to provide an ultimate aim is often more valuable than informing them that nothing can be done straight away.

Counselling

It is probably inappropriate to suggest that nurses should attempt to engage in in-depth counselling activity with patients during an aggressive episode. However, it is entirely appropriate to utilise the basic principles of supportive counselling, provided that they do not increase the degree of mental pressure being experienced by the patient at that time. Additionally, counselling might be indicated and desirable to the patient as part of the solution-focused response during the aggressive incident, for example agreeing to meet for further discussion of a specific identified issue might enable a patient to become calmer by having a reassurance that the issue will be properly discussed at an identified time in the near future.

Diversionary activities

It is important that the use of diversionary activities still takes account of the problem. It is tempting for staff to use diversionary activities as a method of avoiding the problem with no intention of addressing it with the patient at a more appropriate time. The purpose of diversionary activities is to distract the continued escalation of the patient's mood and aggressive behaviour. During the 'distraction period' it is sometimes possible for the patient to begin to calm and begin to engage in the initial stages of problem solving activity. A common example of diversionary activity it to encourage the patient to go for a stroll and a chat in a less stimulating environment. The patient must have an indication that the diversionary activity is likely to be useful in addressing their problem. Diversionary and stimulating activities are part of a therapeutic environment and should occur as part of everyday practice rather than only at difficult times.

Involve others

Aggressive incidents never occur in isolation from other factors, and often an individual or a group of people is targeted with the aggressive behaviour. An important feature of de-escalation should be the notion of informing and involving others who may be able to relate to the patient from a perspective which differs from the immediate conflict situation. Nurses are not always best placed to satisfy a discontented patient (for example, with regard to medication or leave issues). It is reasonable to identify and involve significant or appropriate others in the prevention, de-escalation and management of an aggressive situation.

Safety levels are significantly influenced by the availability of resources and other people. Nurses who are faced with aggressive behaviours when they are alone with a patient are likely to be at a greater level of risk of harm than when other staff members are present. Nurses who knowingly engage with aggressive patients should always ensure that other people know their whereabouts and details of the situation. However, a note of caution is raised concerning the involvement of others. It is possible that the presence of an audience might somehow force the aggressive individual to maintain their level of arousal, or make it difficult for them to change their behaviour for fear of being perceived as 'backing down' or 'losing face'. The presence of other staff should always be non-threatening and 'low key'.

The following clinical example illustrates the positive impact that 'others' can have on a difficult situation.

Case Study: Mr S

Mr S was admitted to the psychiatric intensive care unit (PICU). He was well known to the service due to a number of previous admissions. He presented as hostile and intimidating to staff and patients within the PICU environment. His aggressive presentation was attributed to a relapse in his mental state due to his non-compliance with treatment whilst living independently in the community.

Mr S was known to respond favourably to recommencing treatment at the earliest opportunity and was therefore, prescribed medication. Mr S refused to accept this treatment and negotiation was proving problematic due to a difficulty in establishing a rapport with him. Efforts to discuss the issue of treatment with Mr S appeared to be adding to his already high levels of arousal and hostile behaviour. Several separate attempts to engage Mr S in discussion about the proposed treatment were attempted without success. Subsequently, discussions commenced regarding the possible use of physical restraint to ensure that Mr S received his treatment if he continued to refuse.

Three nurses from other areas were asked to attend the intensive care unit in order to provide additional resources in the event that physical restraint was required. Mr S recognised one of the nurses from his previous admission as she arrived on the ward and a useful dialogue was established. The nurse reminded Mr S that his treatment was important and after a period of time and further negotiation, Mr S agreed to accept it.

Physical intervention

Unfortunately, the aim of involving patients in their care and the concept of fostering autonomy can be compromised when nurses intervene physically. However, it is possible that the mode of intervention, and staff attitudes displayed during any intervention, can significantly minimise the potentially negative effects whilst helping the patient to regain a degree of self-control. Physical interventions to manage aggressive behaviours are considered to be emergency measures that are often viewed as 'last resort' options. However, regardless of their ranking within the range of possible options, it is imperative that whenever physical interventions are employed that they are founded upon care principles. The model of de-escalation proposed by McHugh *et al.* (1995) includes physical restraint as an option that might be necessary as a part of the de-escalation process. The use of physical restraint might not itself de-escalate a patient's expressed anger, but should enable staff to work closely with them to achieve the calming effect in safer conditions.

McHugh *et al.* (1995) assert that de-escalation and problem-solving approaches should be considered key elements of physical restraint. They further suggest that a structured set of skills which gradually return control to the patient are likely to complement the process of de-escalation. In this respect, it is clear that the use and method of physical restraint should be determined by the needs of the situation and the presented behaviour. Physical responses that are based upon inflexible systems are likely to detract from the concept of care and the de-escalation process by their inability to adapt to the changing presentation of the patient who is in the process of calming. Staff require flexible skills, based upon clear principles. By adopting such approaches and skills, it is more likely that staff are able to consistently reflect least restrictive practice in a caring way to patients who are aggressive. This is fundamental to the concept of de-escalation without irreversible damage to the potential for therapeutic alliance.

Appendix 1 shows principles for the use of physical restraint skills in accordance with the standards outlined by the RCNI (1997). These standards and guiding principles are aimed at ensuring that any physical restraint methods employed are not intended or designed to inflict pain or injury. They are intended to satisfy the standard identified by the General Assembly of the United Nations that:

> The restraint of a severely disturbed person is justified as long as the method of restraint does not involve inhumane or degrading treatment. (General Assembly of the United Nations, 1948)

After an aggressive incident

Staff debriefing

The value and importance of staff debriefing is widely acknowledged in the literature. Unfortunately, some nurses view this process as having little practical value, being too time-consuming and intrusive. It is evident that staff support and debriefing occurs naturally within some nursing teams, although informal systems are not necessarily consistent or sufficiently structured always to be effective. It is essential that strategies are developed which have clearly defined lines of progression and boundaries for each stage of the staff care process. Nurses who are expected to work with patients who may exhibit aggressive behaviour are likely to benefit from systems of practice which incorporate opportunities for debriefing into everyday life. It is essential, however, that such opportunities are not provided solely in response to major incidents of aggression. They should ideally provide a regular forum to dissipate the accumulation of feelings and stresses that result from frequent exposure to low-level aggression.

In the past it was not uncommon to see small groups of staff sitting down at the end of their shift to have a cup of tea and talk. This process had many benefits that included opportunities for a degree of initial staff support, staff reassurance, reflection, and consolidation of team working. Unfortunately, it appears that nurses are becoming less likely to be given the facilities or opportunity to engage in such activities during work time.

The incorporation of systems that encourage daily staff team interactions increase staff support and staff care at a 'normal practice' level. Daily nursing team discussion opportunities might be sufficient debriefing for most situations, or might help to identify those nurses or situations that require a more in-depth and structured debriefing or staff counselling. It has been said that hospital patients are well cared for when staff are too.

Reporting and recording

It is important to establish and utilise a system that is able accurately to record incidents of aggression and violence. There are requirements in Health and Safety legislation and the professional need for clinical assessment, audit, research and ultimately maintaining and improving safe services for patients and staff. The UKCC (1998b) indicate that audit, which includes records, can play a vital part in ensuring that quality services are provided to patients. There are numerous models for recording and reporting incidents but the value of such systems relies upon the integrity, objectivity, accuracy and comprehensiveness of the information provided. The potential value of accurate reporting and recording may be lost if it is viewed as a process which is separate from clinical assessment activities. If people are unable to report events in an open and honest manner, for whatever reason, the value of reporting and recording of aggressive incidents is limited.

A model 'Incident Form' might include the following details:

- Identity of the people involved.
- Category of incident.
- Date, time and place of the incident.
- Brief description of the incident (supported by separate 'fact sheets' that are completed by any witnesses to the incident).
- Response to the incident/action taken.
- Details of any injuries sustained by anyone involved in the incident.

- Details of any medical intervention or treatment (including date and time).
- Details of witnesses to the incident.
- Was physical restraint used during the incident (prompts completion of additional form – see below).
- Head of department and administration comments/action.
- Details of any persons absent from work for more than three days as a result of the incident.

Any incident which has necessitated the use of physical skills by staff may also require the completion of a 'Physical Restraint Monitoring Form' (PRMF). A PRMF might include the following:

- Identity of the patient.
- Date and time of day.
- Duration of the application of any physical intervention.
- Details of interventions attempted prior to the physical intervention.
- Reason for the use of the physical intervention.
- Identity of the staff involved.
- Physical methods employed by each person.
- Position that the patient was held in.
- Injuries occurring during the process of physical intervention.
- Subsequent action regarding the management of the patient.
- Use of any protective clothing, e.g. latex gloves.
- Comments regarding difficulties or other relevant points.

Post incident review

Following every incident of aggressive behaviour exhibited by patients, it is important that there is a review of the situation by the staff involved and, wherever appropriate, other staff who know the patient. Such reviews are important because they can help to support and inform the care strategy. Discussions can help provide an accurate picture of the event and clarify the details and important learning points for the patient and staff.

Conclusion

The appropriate management of aggression within health care settings is a highly contentious and difficult issue for nurses. It is better to plan and agree strategies to manage aggressive incidents before they occur. Aggressive behaviour within health care settings is likely to be determined as being hazardous. All reasonable steps should be taken by service managers and clinical staff to develop safe systems of working which reflect evidence based practice for preventing and managing potential or actual aggression in health care settings.

It is important that the clinical practice of nurses who have to work with patients who become aggressive remains founded in ethical principles and the duty of care:

Have a heart that never hardens, a temper that never tires, and a touch that never hurts. (Charles Dickens)

Appendix: Principles of physical restraint skills

- The skills enable carers to care for clients during crisis through teamwork and a co-ordinated approach.
- The skills should be used as acts of care which are combined with de-escalation and problem solving approaches.
- The skills should be complementary to existing care and interactive skills.
- The training programme is designed to challenge practice in order to confirm or change that practice.
- The skills aspire to combine acceptability with effectiveness.
- The skills are client-centred, i.e. client-specific and client-sensitive.
- The skills are designed to take into account the natural range of movement of the client, and to make any movement safe.
- All of the skills concentrate upon the use of technique and positioning rather than strength alone.
- The skills may be included within risk assessment and the planning of care.
- Consistency of individualised client care may be aided by adopting predictable responses to predictable behaviour.
- At times, the appropriate use of these skills may be required in order to fulfil any duty of care. Failure to act positively may result in allegations of negligence.
- The skills allow carers to act positively at times of crisis. They allow a variety of appropriate responses to a situation, which may be proactive, reactive, or last resort.
- The skills incorporate the setting up of good communication and defusing systems that are linked to identified roles.
- The nature and intention of any physical contact is care. The skills offer a multidirectional seamless spectrum of intervention that ranges from touch to holding, to restraint.

References

Blair, D.T. and New, S.A. (1991) Assaultive behavior: know the risks. *Journal of Psychosocial Nursing*, 29 (11), pp. 25–30.

Boettcher, E.G. (1983) Preventing violent behaviour, an integrated theoretical model for nursing. *Perspectives in Psychiatric Care,* 21 (2), pp. 54–8.

Carlisle, D. (1995) Prone to attack. *Nursing Times*, 91 (41), pp. 22–3.

Crichton, J. (1996) Psychiatric inpatient violence. In N. Walker (ed.), *Dangerous People*. Blackwell, Oxford.

Department of Health (1983) The Mental Health Act 1983. HMSO, London.

Department of Health. (1985) Report to the Secretary of State for Social Services concerning the death of Mr Michael Martin at Broadmoor Hospital on 6th July 1984. HMSO, London.

Department of Health (1995) NHS. The Patient's Charter and You. HMSO, London.

Department of Health (1997) NHS. The Patient's Charter. Mental Health Services. HMSO, London.

Department of Health (1999) We Don't Have to Take This: Resource Pack. NHS Zero Tolerance Zone. HMSO, London.

Department of Health and Welsh Office (1999) Code of Practice: Mental Health Act 1983. HMSO, London.

English National Board for Nursing, Midwifery and Health Visiting (1993) Circular 1993/11/GMB: Coping with Violence and Aggression – Prevention and Management. ENB, London.

English National Board for Nursing, Midwifery and Health Visiting (1998) Review of the Year 1997–1998: Working for Excellence in Care. Executive Summary of the Annual Report 1997–1998. ENB, London.

General Assembly of the United Nations (1948) Universal Declaration of Human Rights: Resolution 217(A). United Nations, New York.

Hallberg, I.R., Norberg, A. and Eriksson, S. (1990) A comparison between the care of vocally disruptive patients and that of other residents at psychogeriatric wards. *Journal of Advanced Nursing*, 15, pp. 410–16.

Health and Safety at Work etc. Act (1974), HMSO, London.

Health and Safety Commission (1992a) Management of Health and Safety at Work Regulations. HMSO, London.

Health and Safety Commission (1992b) Workplace Regulations. HMSO, London.

Hodgkinson, P., Hillis, A. and Russell, D. (1984) Assaults on staff in a psychiatric hospital. *Nursing Times*, 80 (16), pp. 44–6.

Home Office Research and Statistics Directorate. (1996) The 1996 British Crime Survey: England and Wales. Information and Publication Group, London.

James, D., Fineberg, N., Shah, A., and Priest, R. (1990) An increase in violence on an acute psychiatric ward. *British Journal of Psychiatry*, 156, 846–52.

Journal of Occupational Health, Safety and Environment (1998) It's dangerous out there. *Journal of Occupational Health, Safety and Environment*, 2 (11), p. 14.

Mackintosh, J.H. (1990) Theories of aggression. In R. Bluglass and P. Bowden (eds), *Principles and Practice of Forensic Psychiatry*. Churchill Livingstone, Edinburgh.

McHugh, A., Wain, I. and West, M. (1995) Handle with care. *Nursing Times*, 91 (6), 62–3.

Mental Health Act Commission (1997) Seventh Biennial Report: 1995–1997. HMSO, London.

Myers, G. and Myers, M. (1985) *The Dynamics of Human Communication*. McGraw-Hill, New York.

Nursing Times (1998) Nursing is a dangerous job and those in the profession demand the right to work in safety. (Editorial – Launch of Stamp Out Violence campaign). *Nursing Times*, 94 (43), p. 3.

Poster, E. and Ryan, J. (1993) At risk of assault. *Nursing Times*, 89 (23), pp. 30–4.

Rosenham, D.L. (1973/1991) On being sane in insane places. In P.J. Barker and S. Baldwin (eds), *Ethical Issues in Mental Health*. Chapman and Hall, London.

Rosenthal, T.L., Edwards, N.B., Rosenthal, R.H. and Ackerman, B.J. (1992) Hospital violence: site, severity, and nurses' preventive training. *Issues in Mental Health Nursing*, 13, 349–56.

Royal College of Nursing (1992) *Seclusion, Control and Restraint*. RCN, London.

Royal College of Nursing (1997) *The Management of Aggression and Violence in Places of Care*. An RCN Position Statement. RCN, London.

Royal College of Nursing (1998) *Dealing with Violence against Nursing Staff*. An RCN Guide for Nurses and Managers. RCN, London.

Royal College of Nursing Institute (1997) *Trainers in the Management of Actual or Potential Aggression*. Code of Professional Conduct and Minimum Training Standards. RCN, London.

Royal College of Psychiatrists (1998) *Management of Imminent Violence*. Clinical Practice Guidelines to Support Mental Health Services. RCP, London.

Rumbold, G. (1993) *Ethics in Nursing Practice*, 2nd edn. Bailliere Tindall, London.

Ryan, J. and Poster, E. (1993) Workplace violence. *Nursing Times*, 89 (48), pp. 38–41.

Schauss, A.G. (1985) The physiological effect of color on the suppression of human aggression:

research on Baker–Miller pink. *International Journal of Biosocial Research*, 7 (2), pp. 55–64.

Shah, A.K. (1993) An increase in violence among psychiatric inpatients: real or apparent? *Medicine, Science and the Law*, 33 (3), 227–30.

Shannon, C. and Weaver, W. (1949) *The Mathematical Theory of Communication*. University of Illinois Press, Illinois.

Stevenson, S. (1991) Heading off violence with verbal de-escalation. *Journal of Psychosocial Nursing and Mental Health Service*, 29 (9), 6–10.

Stirling, C. (1998) Developing a non-aversive intervention strategy in the management of aggression and violence for people with learning disabilities using natural therapeutic holding. *Journal of Advanced Nursing*, 27, pp. 503–9.

Stockwell, F. (1972) *The Unpopular Patient*. RCN, London.

Sullivan, P. (1998) Care and control in mental health nursing. *Nursing Standard*, 13 (15), pp. 42–5.

Tarbuck, P. (1992a) Ethical standards and human rights. *Nursing Standard*, 7 (6), 27–30.

Tarbuck, P. (1992b) Use and abuse of control and restraint. *Nursing Standard*, 6 (52), pp. 30–2.

Topping-Morris, B. (1995) No place for restraint in care. *Nursing Times*, 91 (11), p. 22.

Special Hospitals Service Authority (SHSA) (1993) *Big, Black and Dangerous?* Report of the Committee of Inquiry into the Death in Broadmoor Hospital of Orville Blackwood and a Review of the Deaths of Two Other Afro-Caribbean Patients. SHSA, London.

Trades Union Congress. (1999) *Violent Times*. TUC report on preventing violence at work. Trades Union Congress, London.

UKCC (1992) *Code of Professional Conduct*, 3rd edn. United Kingdom Central Council for Nursing, Midwifery and Health Visiting, London.

UKCC (1996) *Guidelines for Professional Practice*. United Kingdom Central Council for Nursing, Midwifery and Health Visiting, London.

UKCC (1998a) *Guidelines for Mental Health and Learning Disabilities Nursing*. United Kingdom Central Council for Nursing, Midwifery and Health Visiting, London.

UKCC (1998b) *Guidelines for Records and Record Keeping*. United Kingdom Central Council for Nursing, Midwifery and Health Visiting, London.

Walker, Z. and Seifert, R. (1994) Violent incidents in a psychiatric intensive care unit. *British Journal of Psychiatry*, 164, pp. 826–8.

Suicide/self-harm

Shelly Allen and Sarah Beasley

Introduction

Self-harm is undeniably an emotive issue, which evokes a response and opinion arguably in all of us. This is not confined solely to our own beliefs associated with the expression of self-harm but as health care professionals, also relates to the care we offer those requiring the use of services. Self-harm is not synonymous with mental ill health; many people who behave in this way survive life in the community without ever having contact with mental health services. Nor is self-harm solely associated with the group of people often referred to as 'mentally disordered offenders'. Forensic mental health services may not be the most suitable ones to meet the needs of people who self-harm.

What cannot be disputed is that within a population of mentally disordered offenders, some will engage in self-harm and it is reasonable to suggest that this will result in a sense of emotional turmoil and disempowerment for many health care professionals. Given this, it is crucial that clinicians feel supported and are able to deliver a quality service where self-harm may be afforded the same attention as a mental state assessment, or that related to offending behaviour. It is important that information be provided to clinicians to facilitate an informed and sensitive approach, where services attempt to meet the individual's needs rather than the individual attempting to mould themselves around existing provision.

There are no definitive answers to self-harm. The information presented in this chapter is intended to be thought provoking and question the reader's practice, attitude and view of self-harm. In doing so it is envisaged that consideration may be given to a more appropriate service provision and future care delivery within forensic mental health settings. Arnold (1995) reaffirms the importance of a different approach to service delivery:

> Many approaches are based on the theories of academics and clinicians, rather than on what people who themselves self-injure say about their experience and few seem to have asked individuals directly how they understand and interpret their own self-injury, most making their own inferences from clinical experience. (Arnold, 1995, p. 1)

The importance of offering information generated by people who have, and do, engage in self-harm can not be denied. As such the so-called 'user perspective' will be referred to throughout.

Clinical considerations

1. Self-harm is not a psychiatric illness.
2. Many people who self-harm live in the community without input from psychiatric services.
3. Services should be developed to meet the needs of the individual.

Self-harm defined

It is important to offer a definition to facilitate understanding and comprehension of this issue. In the case of self-harm attempts to do this appear contrary to the need for simplicity, and can lead to confusion and misconception.

Many definitions and terms have been used in the literature in an attempt to describe self-harm and how this is qualitatively different to suicide, culturally sanctioned rituals and beliefs or even a 'fad' which may pass in and out of fashion.

There has been a surge of interest in self-harm over the past thirty years, as suggested by Burnham (1969, p. 223) who observed:

> It is remarkable that the literature dealing with this syndrome has been almost nil prior to this year ... Drs Pao, Kafka and Podvoll have substantially increased our written knowledge and understanding of the syndrome and the patients who exhibit it.

Self-harm, however, is not a new phenomenon; its history can be traced throughout the ages in various texts, including the Bible. Favazza and Simeon (1995, p. 185) indicate the passage in the New Testament Gospel of St Mark, Chapter 5, which states that Jesus was requested to help a man who 'night and day, cried and cut himself with stones'. It is perhaps therefore, more accurate to suggest that the more recent surge of interest may relate to distinguished and popular figures who have publicly acknowledged their own episodes of self-injury. Divulgence of such personal experiences may well have raised the profile of self-harm (Hogg, 1996). In addition survivor user-led organisations such as *Survivors Speak Out, The National Self-harm Network* and *For Acceptance and Care to Express Self-Harm (FACES)* have striven to increase awareness and campaign for improved understanding and treatment from health care professionals. Yet despite this there continues to be a lack of agreement within the clinical arena as to what constitutes self-harm.

The first hurdle one is faced with in an attempt to define self-harm is the issue of terminology.

> Deliberate self-harm; deliberate self-injury; deliberate self-poisoning; self-destructive behaviour; self-mutilation; attempted suicide; failed suicide;

non fatal suicide; incomplete suicide; pseudo suicide; para-suicide; self-abusive behaviour and scarification. (Burrow, 1992, p. 139)

What Burrow (1992) refers to as a 'semantic paella' is not merely confined to the above. Further terms include:

Partial suicide; focal suicide; self violence; auto aggression; delicate self cutting; and anti-suicide. (Barstow, 1995, p. 19)

Just as many terms exist, so do many proposed definitions of self-harm. Favazza (1989, p. 137) states that self-mutilation is 'the deliberate self-destruction or alteration of body tissue without conscious suicidal intent'. Bunclark and Adcock (1996) concur with Favazza (1989) in rejecting the notion that self-harm is a failed attempt to kill oneself. Bunclark and Adcock further suggest that although accidental deaths can occur as a result of self-harm, the mortality rate is low compared to that of suicide attempts.

In addition, it is important to stress that terms suggesting self-harm to be a failed attempt by the individual to kill themselves serve little purpose, as they distort the meaning of self-harm and the probable function it serves. The use of such language may also reinforce a negative view of the individual as a failure with an inherent lack of control over their destiny, as illustrated by Babiker and Arnold (1997, p. 6) who state:

There is an important difference between attempted suicide and self-injury and this difference is fairly clear: in attempted suicide the person intends to kill himself, in self-injury the person does not.

The issue of intent in relation to self-harm has been given much consideration and in an attempt to classify self-harm as opposed to attempted suicide, Stengal (1970; cited in Anderson, 1997, p. 1284) stated that 'any deliberate act of self-damage, which the person committing the act cannot be sure to survive' should be classed as attempted suicide. It may be reasonable to suggest that behaviours that interfere with the vital functioning of an individual's body, for example use of ligatures or self-suffocation, are not acts of self-harm but of attempted suicide. Walsh and Rosen (1988, p. 25), however, express concern over assessment of intent in relation to self-harm, stating:

First, the intent of self-mutative acts is inevitably private to its perpetrators. Self-mutilators can never share with us in a direct, immediate way the complex determinants of their acts of self-harm. At best, they can describe after the act what they remember their intent to have been. This memory is, of course, subject to a variety of distortions. Second, the intent of acts of self-harm is often a mystery to the perpetrators themselves.

Despite intent representing an integral part of assessment and subsequent care, this would seem to suggest that intent has little validity, which supports the previously documented view by Kahan and Pattison (1984, p. 30), who stated that:

The concept of 'intent to die' is not useful for classification purposes. This depends upon the subject's report of personal intent, which is subject to many types of psychological defences and distortions.

However, some do consider intent or motivation to be important in the crucial distinction between self-harm and suicide. For instance, Winchel and Stanley (1991, p. 306) state:

Self injurious behaviour is defined as the commission of deliberate harm to one's own body. The injury is done to oneself, without the aid of another person and the injury is severe enough for tissue damage (such as scarring) to result. Acts that are committed with conscious suicidal intent or are associated with sexual arousal are excluded.

Clearly the above indicates the autonomy of the act and excludes sexual preference as a motivational factor behind the behaviour. The suggestions by Kahan and Pattison (1984) and Walsh and Rosen (1988) warrant consideration. It would, nevertheless, seem reasonable to suggest that attempts should be made by the individual, and the health care professional, to identify motivational factors and the reasons for self-harm as this is clearly influential in determining the need for and type of intervention.

In his study of self-harm within a British high security hospital, Burrow (1992) suggested the following operational definition:

Any observable act which resulted in an internal, or external, injury or that was considered likely to cause injury in the fairly immediate future. (Burrow, 1992, p. 140)

When considering what it actually means to the individual who engages in self-harm it is perhaps more informative to consult the user-led literature. The following definition seems an encompassing and useful insight, which aids clarification.

Any ways in which someone might injure, hurt or harm themselves, as a way of coping with unbearable distress. Most of the time these sorts of self-harm are carried out not with the intention of suicide, but on the contrary, as a way of making life bearable, to be able to go on. (Arnold and Magill, 1998, p. 3)

Perhaps as a consequence of the difficulties in attempting to define self-harm, there is also an apparent confusion in relation to the acts themselves. Barstow (1995, p. 19) states that 'there is no general agreement among clinicians and researchers regarding which behaviours should be classed as self-injury/self-mutilation'. Arnold and Magill (1996) and Babiker and Arnold (1997) suggest that 'self-harm is a continuum we all inhabit' (Pembroke, 1998, p. 20). If we accept Pembroke's statement, overwork, sleep deprivation, worry, engaging in dangerous hobbies, self-isolation or remaining in abusive relationships might all be classed as self-harm.

Many of us may recognise aspects of our own behaviour in these descriptions, and whilst some may not entirely endorse that to a degree we all engage in some form of self-harm, it is worthy of consideration in relation to attempts to define the concept.

Clinical considerations

1. A summative definition of self-harm does not exist.
2. Existing definitions can compound confusion of the issue.
3. The crucial difference between attempted suicide and self-harm must be acknowledged.

'Self-harmers' – a minority group

Tantum and Whitaker (1992) state that at least 1 in 600 adults seek hospital treatment as a result of self-harm. This figure does not account for those who self-harm and do not receive treatment. It may be then that this figure is an underestimation of the actual prevalence of self-harm. American authors Favazza and Conterio (1988) estimate that a prevalence of 750 per 100 000 population per year seems reasonable. These authors further add that this figure may increase to 1800 per 100 000 people who self-mutilate if it were confined to the peak incidence age of 15 to 35 years (Favazza and Conterio, 1988). This would suggest that the exact number of people who engage in self-harm is not known, which to an extent is perhaps explained by the suggestion that to date no studies have been carried out in the general population (Arnold and Magill, 1996), although the *Guardian* newspaper (12 May 1998) reported 'an estimated 0.75% of the population – 1 in 130 people are active self injurers'. Melville and House (1998) claim that self-harm may be one of the top five reasons for acute medical admissions in the United Kingdom.

It must be acknowledged that self-harm is often private to the individual and carried out in secret (Babiker and Arnold, 1997). Clearly as with many acts which are deemed socially unacceptable and stigmatised, people engaging in self-harm may only be discovered unintentionally, for instance if hospital treatment is required.

Even if an anonymous survey were conducted, people may not wish to disclose self-harm. Thus many incidents are not included in estimations of prevalence and it seems likely, therefore, that self-injury is far more common than is generally recognised (Arnold and Magill, 1996). Whilst true prevalence and incidence cannot be determined, however, health care professionals are likely to work with individuals displaying self-harm. As Burrow (1994) states, 'All nurses will, at some time in their career, come into contact with patients who appear to damage themselves voluntarily' (Burrow, 1994, p. 382). Such contact is not merely confined to mental health nurses, nor indeed nurses *per se*. So it is important that through education, the dissemination of research findings and consultation with user groups, attempts are made to dispel misconceptions, and improve and develop services to meet the needs of the individual.

Clinical considerations

1. Prevalence and incidence of self-harm are underestimated.
2. To date, a study of the general population has not been conducted.
3. Self-harm occurs in all walks of life.

'Self-harmers': attention seeking?

In terms of psychiatric diagnosis, personality disorder and self-harm are often associated and these individuals may be perceived as difficult (Fraser and Gallop, 1993). In some instances this judgement may be made even before there is any contact between the individual and service provider.

Burrow (1994) states that health care staff either view self-harm as symptomatic of wider psychological illness or as a characteristic of helpless pathetic isolated people, not in control of themselves. This polarisation of opinion in relation to self-harm is further described by Allen (1995), who refers to some practitioners as the so-called 'counsel of despair' who argue that people with personality disorders are incurable and that anyone who listens to them sympathetically indulges them and reinforces their self-harm behaviour. Conversely Allen (1995) also de-sensitises the 'naive therapeutic optimist' who advocates the belief that people who self-harm desperately need therapy and that once their appalling history has been talked through the problem will go away. Favazza (1989) states that although self-harm is prevalent, attempts to understand it have been influenced by negative social attitudes. As Allen (1995) has also suggested, 'The range of emotions evoked, including panic, hopelessness, anger and even hate, makes a consistent, therapeutic response very difficult to achieve. As a result, people who harm themselves often receive a poor service when they turn to professional systems for help' (Allen, 1995, p. 243).

Yet in some cultures self-harm is an acceptable activity and represents adolescent initiation rites during which pain and mutilation must be endured (Favazza and Conterio, 1988). It has also been equated with a tradition whereby Shamans would endure their bodies being symbolically dismembered and reconstructed, emerging as wiser and healthier people capable of healing (Eliade, 1975).

Health care professionals, not just nurses, inherently wish to assist those who seek help. This extends, in the case of forensic mental health care, to those whose mental health problems have contributed to their committing a crime. In these circumstances there is an expectation that care and services will be made available with a non-judgemental approach. It does appear, however, that society, including many health care professionals, view self-harm as generally unacceptable. Burrow (1994, p. 383) makes the observation that:

> At worst, it may be considered that the perversity of enduring suffering and disfigurement defies rational explanation and indicates a bad, manipulative, attention-seeking personality. It is small wonder that nursing staff are inadequately prepared for clinical encounters that seem

to run counter to the perception that they function to assist the deserving sick.

It may be reasonable to suggest that this lack of preparation may influence some treatment offered by professionals and the consequent effect this has on the individual. Pembroke (1994, p. 36) states that:

Going to accident and emergency had become a form of self-harm. The judgement of the staff confirmed that I really was the lowest form of life and reinforced every negative feeling I had ever had about myself.

This judgemental attitude displayed by health care staff is concurred with by McLaughlin (1994, p. 1112), who observes that:

Physical illness such as myocardial infarction and cerebro-vascular accident elicit positive attitudes in nurses...patients who are admitted following an overdose elicit particularly negative attitudes in nurses.

Gibbs (1990) indicates that self-harm is often seen as unwelcome extra work in environments where staff perceive themselves to be under pressure.

Pembroke's (1994) observation that when professionals had shown compassion and respect following self-injury this increased the individual's self-worth and helped to delay further acts of self-injury is reassuring. It is therefore comforting to note that not all professionals stand in condemnation of those who self-harm. People who are often reluctant to use services, be they accident and emergency or related to mental health, should be provided with effective care which does not compound this reluctance further. As practitioners we should be mindful of the warning from Allen (1995, p. 246) against the 'tendency to believe that any kind of counselling, even from an untrained, inexperienced helper, is better than none'.

Authors including Ghodse *et al.* (1986), Bailey (1994) and Hemmings (1997) have endorsed the need for practitioners to access education. Similarly McGaughey and Harrison (1995) indicate the importance of further training and education to develop professionals' understanding, which would also assist in changing the negative attitudes that at present appear to be a major contributor to ineffective care. In an attempt to encourage such developments acknowledgement must be given to the work of individuals such as Christine Hogg and Maureen Burke, both based in the Northwest of England, who have striven for the inclusion of self-harm in academic study, in an attempt to redress the lack of preparation described by Burrow (1994).

In addition, support and supervision are crucial to the maintenance of effective practice. Even the most dedicated member of staff working with an individual who engages in self-harm can become disheartened on occasion. As Arnold and Magill (1996, p. 8) state:

Working with people who self injure inevitably raises many difficult issues and feelings...self injury naturally arouses many uncomfortable feelings, however professional we are. We would have to be inhuman not to experience strong reactions.

However, it is important to recognise that strong reactions are attributed to frustration rather than condemnation of the person. It was in response to recognition for the need to support practitioners working with people who self-harm that the Northwest Self-Injury Interest Group comprised of health care professionals was established. This led to the subsequent formation of the Self-Injury Group at Reaside Clinic, where clinicians are encouraged to attend the group for peer support, education and discussion.

Self-Injury Group philosophy

The Self-Injury Group (SIG) at Reaside Clinic was established due to a perceived need to develop and educate staff in the pursuit of enhanced practice with individuals who self-harm. This was not the sole aim of the group, as it was also recognised that colleagues must support each other and share experiences. It was on this basis that initial endeavours were made to establish the group. Having achieved this, the general philosophy can be broadly summarised in the following manner.

- Whilst there are a core group of members, the SIG does not demand fixed membership. Participants are encouraged to attend the group and any meetings thereafter as their interest or need dictates.
- The group may be used to facilitate expression of concerns, worries or frustrations. Such contribution is welcome and as a group the SIG members will attempt to support and share pertinent experiences with others and dispel myths associated with self-harm where necessary.
- SIG believes that individuals who self-harm have the right to be treated with the same respect and dignity we would afford ourselves. People who self-harm should be helped to express what they perceive their needs to be. These should be recognised and valued, with efforts being made to achieve them where possible.
- It is crucial whilst accepting the constraints of working with individuals within a medium secure unit (MSU), that residents be cared for in conjunction with their needs. These should continually be assessed and the consequent care implemented and evaluated regularly. This should facilitate the appropriate level of therapeutic intervention without inappropriate infringement on the individual's privacy and in conjunction with the maintenance of a safe environment for them and others.
- Those who engage in self-harm should be regarded in a non-judgemental and professional manner by those involved in their care.
- Whilst it is appreciated that staff may become frustrated and disillusioned when caring for individuals who self-harm, the group advocate that expression of such emotions should be in the appropriate setting.
- Just as clinicians must listen to those individuals who self-harm, it is also important as health care professionals that we allow ourselves the opportunity to express our own concerns and worries and expect to be received by others in a non-judgemental manner. This we believe is crucial in maintaining a therapeutic relationship with our service users, providing high standards of care and promoting good working relations with colleagues from all disciplines.

- It is recognised that practice must be based on sound research findings. As a group it is not only through the collection of relevant research and its subsequent critique that we endorse this, but also as a result of individual members completing research work relating to self-harm.

Case study A

Now in her early twenties, person A has been resident in secure provision for more than two years. She describes an unhappy childhood with parental disharmony and alleged abuse.
Frequently feeling bored, a truant from school and regularly misusing illicit substances, A lived with her grandparents with relationships within the family remaining strained.
Many acts of self-harm have been recorded during A's admission, for instance during a three month period eighty incidents were reported, including scratches, ligature use and insertion of foreign bodies.
Through discussion and exploration of the motivation behind these acts of self-harm she has disclosed and dealt with many issues which caused her acute distress, such as her index offence, body image, and abusive relationships.

Clinical considerations

1. Education for the multiprofessional team is crucial.
2. Clinical supervision must be available.
3. Practitioners must be trained to work therapeutically with people who self-harm.
4. Negative attitudes must be challenged.

Diagnosis and self-harm

Self-harm is not a diagnosis, although it does feature as one criterion for certain types of mental disorder. Repeated self-mutilation is one symptom of borderline personality disorder specified in DSM III R (Favazza and Conterio, 1988; Tantam and Whitaker, 1992), as well as of both narcissistic and histrionic disorders of personality (Favazza and Conterio, 1988; Konicki and Schultz, 1989). The appropriateness of this has been debated both within the clinical arena and the literature. As Johnstone (1997) states:

> The argument is circular: 'Why does this woman cut herself? Because she has borderline personality disorder. How do you know she has borderline personality disorder? Because she cuts herself.' (Johnstone, 1997, pp. 23–4)

This statement is important and calls into question the validity of using self-harm as a diagnostic criterion.

It has been estimated that 1 per cent of all adults and 50 per cent of prisoners (Favazza and Conterio, 1988) are thought to have an antisocial personality disorder. Yet in a study conducted by Virkkunen (1976, cited in Winchel and Stanley, 1991), within a prison population, the author found that of 80 inmates half indulged in self-harm whilst the other half did not, despite all fulfilling the criteria for antisocial personality disorder. Likewise in a population of psychiatric inpatients who self harmed, personality disorder was not diagnosed more frequently than in a control group of non-psychotic in-patients (Gardner and Gardner, 1975, cited in Tantum and Whitaker (1992).

Aside from what may be considered clear limitations to using self-harm as a diagnostic criterion, Tantum and Whitaker (1992, p. 454) warn of the possibility that 'too often further inquiry into the reasons for the behaviour, in particular into the situational determinants of self wounding, stops once a diagnosis is made'.

It is not only this that warrants consideration, but also the consequences of diagnoses, which can be far reaching, as described by Pembroke (1994, p. 46):

> Labels tend to be assigned to individuals whose patterns of distress do not 'fit' into any of the other psychiatric categorisations . . . 'anti-social', 'deviant', 'difficult' . . . all lead to the diagnosis of personality disorder . . . if the clinician doesn't know what category to put the patient into, standby dustbin diagnoses are given: personality disorder, behavioural disorder.

Harrison concurs with this latter view (1995, p. 9) when she describes herself as a 'survivor of deliberate self-harm':

> The hysterical, neurotic woman image follows us through our notes making it feel as if our credibility is at stake any future appointments for whatever problem become clouded with a degree of prior judgement.

Pembroke (1994, p. 35) develops this observation further, stating that 'calling me neurotic transforms the act of self-harm to "attention seeking", while "psychotic" changes self-harm to "understandable"'.

Borderline personality disorder and self-harm often attracts the label of the unpopular patient (Gallop *et al.*, 1993; Burrow, 1994; Loughrey *et al.*, 1997). Miller (1994, pp. 160–1) states:

> Perhaps the most damaging aspect for the client who is diagnosed as borderline is that she has been labelled as someone who is not nice to therapists or to anyone else trying to help her . . . it signals to other clinicians that the client is difficult or even unmanageable and has a poor prognosis.

We must urge consideration to be given when working with people who self-harm that, 'when clinicians adopt negative attitudes or opinions toward a client deemed problematic or unpopular, this can have a domino effect on others working with that client' (Hillis and McClelland, 1998, p. 29).

Hillis and McClelland (1998) further propose that pessimistic views projected by practitioners may lead to the client rejecting the clinician or adopting some of the negative attributes and absorbing or internalising feelings of unpopularity. Clearly this is far from conducive to effective care.

Clinical considerations

1. Self-harm is not a psychiatric diagnosis.
2. Diagnoses, if required, should be given with care and the risk of labelling acknowledged.

Gender and self-harm

Johnstone (1997, pp. 23–4) used the female pronoun when describing the circular argument which revolves around diagnosis and self-harm. Many studies of self-harm generally appear to identify their sample population as being predominantly female; this gender association is perhaps reinforced by the crucial work undertaken by women from survivor groups, service users and within academic and clinical settings.

Favazza and Conterio (1988) found that of 250 respondents to a questionnaire sent as a result of a televised programme on self-harm, 96 per cent were female. The authors do, however, suggest that this may have been due to the television programme's audience, rather than the existence of an association between self-harm and women. Miller (1994, p. 5) offers this statement in relation to gender and self-harm:

> Men who have been traumatised in childhood are likely to inflict on others what was done to them; they are socialised to act aggressively and to fight back rather than to allow someone to harm or humiliate them. Women are socialised not to fight back; allowing themselves to be hurt or humiliated is far more socially acceptable than being aggressive or violent toward others. Although some women become abusers themselves, it is much more likely that female victims of childhood trauma will inflict pain on themselves. Men act out. Women act out by acting in.

This view is advocated by others, such as Pembroke (1991, p. 30), who believes that 'a women's worth is gauged by her appearance; that expressions of anger and assertion are not easily tolerated'.

Hawton *et al.* (1997) found that in Oxford the biggest rise in self-harm over 10 years was within 15–24-year-old males, although more incidents of self-harm were attributed to females every year. This pattern of repetitive self-harm in females appears evident in populations of mentally disordered offenders. In a study of self-harm in a British special hospital, Burrow (1992) identifies a population where females represent the minority (30 per cent) yet account for 64 per cent of self-harm incidents. Similarly, Garner and Butler (1994) found that roughly equal numbers of male and female patients engaged in self-harm in a Regional Secure Unit, although more incidents were attributed to the female group.

Garner *et al.* (1996) discovered that during a nine-month period between 1993 and 1994 seven females were responsible for 77.5 per cent of all incidents of self-harm, despite their total proportion of inpatient population during the specified study period being just 12 per cent.

Beasley (1999) observed that patients of female gender who self-harmed accounted for 6 per cent of the inpatient population but were involved in 79 per cent of self-harm incidents. As a result of such research findings a pattern appears to emerge whereby women, a minority group within secure provision, account for the majority of recorded incidents of self-harm. Burrow (1992) attempted to explain the reasons for this phenomenon within the population of mentally disordered offenders by proposing the view of Casale (1989) that positive discrimination exists in favour of keeping women out of prison. He further suggests that this could explain the more concentrated population of disturbed women in special hospitals.

Burrow (1992) suggests that female deviance is more readily medicalised, but concludes that none of these suggestions alone is an adequate explanation for the over-representation of females in his study. The issue is more complex than merely suggesting that self-harm is a predominantly female activity. Indeed, some have stated that self-harm is equally prevalent in both genders (Simpson, 1975; Weissman, 1975; Pattison and Kahan, 1983; Hawton and Catalan, 1987; Clarke and Whitaker, 1998). Tantum and Whitaker (1992) suggest that self-wounding is more prevalent in men than women but that more females receive psychological treatment. Further to this, White *et al.* (1999) found that self-harm among the male population of a Regional Secure Unit was greater than previously reported and in some instances exceeded that documented in relation to women. White *et al.* (1999) also reported the nature of self-harm in men to be similar to that of women. However, the Mental Health Foundation (1997) indicate that males adopt more violent and non-negotiable methods of self-harm than their female counterparts, thus culminating in a higher incidence of completed suicides. This is in keeping with Barnes (1982, p. 466), who notes that, 'although women injure themselves more frequently than do men, men actually kill themselves twice as often as do women'.

Babiker and Arnold (1997, p. 42) suggest that whilst feminist movements have 'given a voice to the experience of women in relation to self injury' there is no 'real parallel to account for men's experience'. To an extent this may explain the association seemingly readily made between women and self-harm.

Females may or may not be at a higher risk of self-harm than males; there does however appear to be a qualitative difference in relation to gender. This being that females are more likely to engage in repetitive acts whilst male attention is focused on more violent forms of self-harm.

Clinical considerations

1. Females and males self-harm but there appears to be a qualitative difference.
2. Male self-harm appears to have increased over the past decade.

Beginning to self-harm

Favazza and Conterio (1988, 1989) indicate the mean age of people who self-harm is 28 years. However, the onset of self-harm is considerably younger; the literature tends to suggest this to be during adolescence (Pattison and Kahan, 1983; Favazza and Conterio, 1988, 1989; Arnold,

1995). Beasley (1999) further supported this and showed that some had their first episode of self-harm aged 14 years. Walsh and Rosen (1988) indicate adolescence to be confusing and difficult to come to terms with. It is also a time when Babiker and Arnold (1997) state independence is established and some adolescents may feel increasingly isolated and rejected by those who are their prime providers of care, which may contribute to the expression of self-harm. However, despite knowledge pertaining to the onset of self-harm, the causal factors remain elusive despite many different approaches being taken.

Russ (1992, p. 77) offers a review of biological perspectives in relation to people diagnosed with borderline personality disorder who self-harm, and concludes that, 'at present, there is no conclusive evidence that specific biological mechanisms are associated with self injurious behaviour in patients with borderline personality disorder'.

Some authors have considered the possibility of learning theory in the perpetuation of self-harm, for instance Walsh and Rosen (1988) suggest this as an explanation for the spread of self-harm within institutions. Sakinofsky and Roberts (1990) discuss the effects of reinforcement and self-perpetuating behaviour in relation to the continuation of self-harm. Such suggestions, however, are not an entirely adequate explanation for the onset of self-harm. In the pursuit of this some authors have studied the possible influence of traumatic experiences in childhood and their relationship to the development of self-harm. Physical abuse is one aspect of this discussed in the literature (Van der Kolk *et al.*, 1991; Faye, 1995). Favazza and Conterio (1989) found that 54 per cent of their community sample described their childhood as miserable whilst 16 per cent reported physical abuse as children.

It has been suggested, however, that many people with mental health problems have a history of childhood trauma which suggests that these experiences are not specifically related to a particular behaviour (Russ, 1992). Whilst this may be the case, it is interesting to note that some studies have emphasised the degree of trauma involved as paramount in the development of later self-harm. Van der Kolk *et al.* (1991) suggested that severe histories of separation and neglect contributed further to the continuation of self-destructive behaviour.

In a comparison between prisoners who self-harm or attempt suicide and other prisoners, Liebling (1995) found that although the presence of family violence between the two groups was similar, it was the degree to which it was reported which was most striking in the group that self-harmed. These people were more likely to indicate frequent violence, multiple family breakdown and local authority placement as a result of family problems. In addition they were more likely to report sexual abuse, particularly the female prisoners.

The experience of childhood sexual abuse amongst people who later self-harm is almost overwhelming in the literature. Powell and Wyatt (1988, p. 106) define child sexual abuse as, 'occurring before the subject was 18 years old: involving intentional and unambiguous sexual behaviour of a physical (rather than merely verbal) nature: and involving a perpetrator who was either at least 5 years older than the victim or who used some type of coercion to secure participation'. Favazza and Conterio (1989) found that

17 per cent of their sample reported sexual abuse as children and further that 29 per cent reported both sexual and physical abuse. In a random community sample, Romans *et al.* (1995) found that childhood sexual abuse and later incidents of self-harm were linked. The authors further state that whilst a minority of sexually abused women reported self-harm, almost all the women who self-harmed had a history of sexual abuse in childhood.

As in Liebling (1995), Romans *et al.* (1995) discuss the importance of the degree of abuse, stating that the more intrusive and frequent the sexual abuse the more strongly it was associated with later self-harm. A correlation is also suggested between age and severity of abuse. The younger the child the more severe and persistent the self-harm (Babiker and Arnold, 1997). Favazza and Conterio (1988) rightly indicate the diversities involved which make it impossible to make a unitary aetiological formulation for people who harm themselves. However, Bunclark and Adcock (1996) offer a summary of the possible spiral of the individual into self-harm, stating that repeated traumatic experiences damage the person's concept of self. The realisation as the individual grows then gives way to guilt and blame leading to feelings of worthlessness. Compounded by repeated experiences of being ignored, the individual stops expressing emotions in the socially accepted way and self-harm may result. This is succinctly described by Babiker and Arnold (1997), 'for most individuals self-injury seems to be associated with extremely difficult and distressing life experiences, often beginning in childhood' (p. 57). Incidence of self-harm among young offenders is significant (Thornton, 1990; Winkler, 1992). Adolescents within secure settings were often found to injure themselves for the first time, citing bullying (Liebling, 1992), a desire to escape a situation, overwhelming feelings of claustrophobia and loss of family as reasons for doing so (Inch *et al.*, 1995).

In terms of adult experiences that may precipitate self-harm it has been suggested that there is a dearth of research (Babiker and Arnold, 1997), although Arnold (1995) found that the nature of these experiences was similar to those in childhood, citing sexual abuse, abusive relationships and lack of support/communication as significant factors. Little attention appears to have been given to older adults and self-harm. Babiker and Arnold (1997) have indicated their uncertainty over whether self-harm declines with age. They further suggest that social stigma may be experienced by older people and thus impinge upon a desire to report self-harm. In conjunction with the loss of the roles of mother, wife and carer, older women may feel isolated which in turn may impact on self-esteem. However, it has also been suggested that a decrease in self-harm with age may be associated with emotional maturity and rejection of social pressures.

Clinical considerations

1. Self-harm often begins in adolescence.
2. No conclusive evidence exists to suggest why people self-harm in the first instance.

Self-harm and ethnicity

The relationship between ethnicity and self-harm appears to be a neglected area. This not only applies to the apparent lack of specific studies aimed at examining ethnicity and self-harm, but also extends to a disregard of such information in some samples. Within the available literature Soni Raleigh and Balarajan (1992) examined suicide and self-burning among Indians and West Indians in England and Wales, which included information concerning self-harm. The authors state that the causes of self-harm among people of Indian origin abroad are not dissimilar to those in their country of origin. These include interpersonal disputes, though rarely the result of racial prejudice, or migration, although they concede that the latter may exacerbate the pressure experienced by the individual. Merrill and Owens (1988) found that self-poisoning amongst Asian and West Indian males of all ages and that of older females was under-represented. However, it should be acknowledged that census information available at that time classified individuals by place of birth rather than ethnic group which may influence the results of this study. In a study conducted by Favazza and Conterio (1989), the sample consisted of 97 per cent Caucasian females, the explanation suggested for this finding being due to a sampling artefact and that the clinical impression of most workers suggests no racial differences. Even so, Wilkins and Coid (1991) found that 93 per cent of women who self-harmed in Holloway prison were Caucasian. Similarly Allen (1997) found that 97 per cent of women residing in a forensic mental health setting who self-harmed were white. It should be acknowledged that the number of black and Asian women in the study was comparatively small and may not be representative.

Clinical considerations

1. There is a dearth of information pertaining to ethnicity and self-harm.
2. To tailor services appropriately more attention is required to this neglected aspect of self-harm.

Function of self-harm

The function of self-harm is undeniably multifaceted and individual. Favazza and Conterio (1988) suggest that self-mutilation may provide a rapid if short lived relief from episodes of depersonalisation, severe anxiety, intense anger, depression, hallucinations, perceived external or internal flaws, racing thoughts and rapidly fluctuating emotions, boredom and stimulus deprivation and feelings of loneliness, emptiness and insecurity.

Barstow (1995) indicates the use of self-harm in tension reduction and suggests that by inducing physical pain the individual may reduce the emotional distress they are experiencing. This was also supported by Rosenthal *et al.* (1972, cited in Burrow, 1992). Allen (1995) suggests that self-harm allows the individual a release of emotion, and on occasion acts as a form of self-punishment. Harrison has stated:

I began hurting myself because it made sense of the confusion and pain I experienced but was unable to voice. Sometimes I would hurt myself to prove I existed. The sight of blood was exciting; it was something I could control. Cutting or scratching myself with twigs or whatever I could find mattered a lot to me. I could care for my wounds, look after them and make them better. This eased for a while my emotional pain. (Harrison, 1995, p. 91)

Clinical considerations

1. The function of self-harm is multifaceted and individual.
2. It is not simply attention-seeking behaviour and this view is counterproductive to effective care.

Self-harm activity

Favazza and Conterio (1989) found cutting was the most prevalent form of activity, with results indicating it was a method employed by 72 per cent of their sample. Burrow (1992), in his study in a high security hospital inpatient population found head banging to be the most common form of self-harm, implicated in 28.6 per cent of incidents while cutting accounted for 26 per cent. Forty-two per cent of this sample engaged in poly-injurious behaviour, which the author defines as three or more forms of activity.

Many studies (for example, Hemkendries, 1992; Garner *et al.*, 1996; Allen, 1997; Hardie, 1998; Beasley, 1999) report that self-harm activity is significantly increased in the evening. There is no definitive explanation as to why this should be but some authors have offered speculative hypotheses, such as biological changes in the body (Hardie, 1998), a fear of going to sleep (Hemkendries, 1992) or because the evening has been associated with abuse in childhood (Beasley, 1999).

Case study: B

At 30 years old, person B has not lived in the community since she was 15, having spent the intervening years in prison and secure psychiatric facilities. A difficult childhood culminated in B being prosecuted for assault. Prior to this there was a criminal history that consisted mainly of convictions for interpersonal violence. Self-harm was present from the age of 9, when an alleged rape had occurred. Periodically B has refrained from self-harm, which has taken many forms during admission including laceration, insertion of foreign bodies, self-strangulation and overdose. Many issues have been explored in relation to her childhood experiences and the consequences of residing in institutions for such a prolonged period of time. The self-harm has become less life-threatening and she has also demonstrated a desire to return to life in the community. This has enabled her to rekindle relationships and explore the other options open to her. This has been a gradual process with safety and support being offered in an attempt to prevent feelings of abandonment which have so often previously resulted in periods of acute distress.

Clinical considerations

1. Environmental factors within hospitals/units often influence the method of self-harm due to accessibility.
2. The method of self-harm is not indicative of intent or motivational factors.
3. Identifying patterns of self-harm activity may be useful to the individual.

Contagion and self-harm

Some have considered the effect of contagion in relation to self-harm, particularly when considering the place of specialised units designed to cater for this group of people. Morse and Mitcham (1997) suggest the most common example of contagion to be yawning, whilst in specific relation to self-harm, it has been suggested this is 'a sequence in which one individual inflicts self-injury and then others in the immediate environment imitate the behaviour' (Walsh and Rosen, 1988, p. 79). Debate exists in the literature as to whether contagion actually exists. Ross and McKay (1979, p. 62) suggest that epidemics of self-injurious behaviour are 'more metaphorical than actual' suggesting that anecdotal evidence influences perceptions. However authors such as Walsh and Rosen (1988), Favazza (1996), Garner and Butler (1994), Taiminen *et al.* (1998) and Beasley (1999) have found statistical evidence to confirm the contagious nature of self-harm.

Garner and Butler (1994) found in a Regional Secure Unit that, following an incident of self-harm, there was an 80 per cent chance of another incident occurring on the same day, a 45 per cent chance of two incidents on the same day and 10 per cent of three. Furthermore, in the same Regional Secure Unit, Beasley (1999) found that up to nine patients were involved in clusters of incidents occurring over a five-day period. Self-harm should not been seen merely in relation to the act itself but in a holistic manner which considers the individual person and not the self-harm in isolation. Therapeutic aims should be realistic and achievable; they should not set the individual up to fail by always setting goals that may never be achieved.

Clinical considerations

1. Evaluation of therapeutic input should not be based on a the number of self-harm incidents.
2. The therapeutic aim should individual, achievable and realistic.

Caring for people who self-harm

It should be appreciated that many people who self-harm do not receive hospital treatment. Romans *et al.* (1995) found that only two-thirds of a community sample had been in contact with a mental health professional. Clinical observation and the literature indicate that within a forensic mental health setting self-harm does occur, and for some patients, frequently and in a persistent way. As such, our duty of care demands that we have an awareness of appropriate and informed strategies in the pursuit of effective treatment. Many approaches used in an effort to eliminate the incidence of self-harm have proved futile. Favazza and Conterio (1988) identified that, of their respondents, 14 per cent stated that hospital treatment had helped a lot, 44 per cent a little, whilst a substantial proportion of 42 per cent stated they felt in-patient intervention had not helped at all. It could be that it is the health professional's approach which is ineffectual; realistic interventions are needed. Bunclark and Adcock (1996, p. 702) suggest that the aim of a tolerant approach would 'not expect immediate elimination of the behaviour, but offer support and gradually enable the self-harming individual to find alternative coping strategies'.

The practice of continually observing a person who is intent on self-harm has been discussed in the literature. In a study conducted by Shugar and Rehaluk (1990), 43 of 102 subjects were continually observed due to a potential risk or actual self-harm. In this Canadian sample in a psychiatric teaching hospital, five clinical factors were shown to predict the use of continuous observation. These were history of self-harm, involuntary status, being of social class IV or V, a history of violence to property, and female gender. Shugar and Rehaluk (1990) further suggest that whilst continuous observation may be effective as a brief management strategy during acute phases, after 72 hours it often becomes problematic and cost-ineffective.

In practice periods of continuous observation for longer than three days do occur. This may be degrading for the individual and therefore counterproductive, and can also be tiring for those carers. They may become a reluctance to discontinue for fear of the consequences, which merely perpetuates anxiety and increases the length of time of intense observation. Practice guidance produced by the Department of Health (1999b, p. 2) states:

> observing a patient who is deeply distressed and potentially suicidal is one of the most difficult and demanding tasks that a nurse can undertake calling for empathy and engagement combined with a readiness to act. Whereas most nursing interventions are intended to help patients achieve their own goals observation is deliberately designed to frustrate the patient's aims. Consequently patients who are observed may be very angry with staff, or may experience the process as custodial and dehumanising.

It is recommended in these guidance notes that decisions over observation levels are made jointly between nursing and medical staff. This should be founded on accurate assessment of risk based on past and present information, gathered from clinical notes, the patient, their family and significant others, and observations of the patient.

The Mental Health Act 1983 Code of Practice (Department of Health, 1999a, p. 101) states, 'Patients must be protected from harming themselves when the drive to self-injury is a result of mental disorder for which they are receiving care and treatment'. There exists an ethical dilemma in relation to this guidance. Whilst a duty of care cannot be denied, how therapeutic are restraint and prevention from self-harm given that this may be the only coping mechanism available to the individual in that instance? Clearly such issues need careful consideration, with clinicians gaining support and guidance from managers in relation to strategies and policies aimed at managing self-harm.

Hillbrand (1992), Swinton and Hopkins (1996) and Beasley (1999) found that a high proportion of incidents of aggression towards others were attributable to patients who also engaged in repetitive acts of self-harm. This contradicts the notion that self-harm derives from a source of anger directed inwardly, suggested by authors such as Arnold (1997). However, it should be stressed that aggression towards others may be confined to a particular population and cannot be generalised to others who self-harm. It may also be fair to suggest that management strategies within secure provision may exacerbate this aggression, for instance if patients are to be protected from harming themselves they may react badly to the well-meaning intentions of the health care professional set on preventing them from self-harm. Pembroke (1991) suggests that physical restraint, used as a strategy to protect the patient from further harm being inflicted, may exacerbate frustration and lead to more extensive injuries. Favazza (1996) suggests that persons who are frustrated are more likely to demonstrate aggression (Dollard *et al.*, 1939).

Medication may be administered to the distressed individual as a method employed during acute episodes. Burrow's (1992) study indicated this as the most frequent intervention used. Whilst it may be used in an effort to maintain a safe environment, it is a short-term strategy whose efficacy should not be overestimated. Nor should it be used in isolation as the precipitating factor leading to self-harm will often not have been identified or dealt with.

The need for thorough assessment, conducted by the individual and clinician, is of paramount importance. Bunclark and Adcock (1996) discuss the need for a detailed history to be obtained, including all previous methods of self-harm and the consequent medical intervention used. They further state it is important to document whether and how help was sought and the frequency of such incidents. The individual's social, psychological and medical needs should be included as well as information regarding any previous suicide attempts. This will help planning of future interventions by the individual and professional, as advocated by Williams and Morgan (1994).

Hawton (1990) states that based on a thorough history, interventions can then be explored with the individual. He further advocates the use of relaxation techniques to counter tension, ventilation and physical exercise as a distraction, physical contact with a confidante, assertiveness training and cognitive methods to explore what provokes the expression of self-harm.

The need for multi-professional working in relation to self-harm is advocated by Kapur *et al.* (1999, p. 172), who state, 'multidisciplinary approaches to assessment of deliberate self-harm have several advantages: the range of available interventions is increased; skills can be shared; administrative efficiency and speed of response may be increased, and the team approach helps maintain morale in a service dealing with a challenging patient group.' They further suggest that strategies could be developed around planning groups and clear hospital policies which are 'major determinants of standards of patient care, and have an important part to play in improving care of deliberate self-harm'.

It is important to recognise the importance of multidisciplinary working but also to maintain an appreciation that too many professionals directly involved with one individual may be counterproductive. A balance must be achieved. Practice guidelines have been developed by the members of Self-Injury Group at Reaside Clinic. These are given in Box 5.1.

Box 5.1 Guidelines for good practice

Attitude toward individuals who self-injure
- Care should be delivered with an empathetic attitude.
- Labelling and stigmatising is not acceptable.
- A professional and consistent approach should be maintained.

Care of individuals who self-injure
- A safe environment should be maintained for the patient and clinician.
- Treatment and first aid should be administered as required, maintaining dignity and respect.
- Treatment of physical injuries should be according to severity rather than origin.
- Each incident should be managed individually, in conjunction with full assessment of the individual and their needs.
- A holistic approach should be adopted, incorporating wider issues pertinent to the individual, without solely focusing on self-injury.

Issues relating to care delivery
- Care packages should be evidence based.
- A collaborative approach to care should be adopted between the patient and clinician.
- An option to be considered in the planning of care which will support clinicians and assure the quality of care delivery, is to establish a group approach, led by an identified key worker to assess, plan, implement and review care, in liaison with the patient and clinical team.
- All members of the care group should meet at regular intervals.
- A team approach to care should be emphasised to the individual, being informed that information divulged will be shared, in confidence, with other members of the clinical team.

Issues relating to the clinician
- A forum should exist, such as the Self-Injury Group, where clinicians can reflect upon their practice, sharing experiences and resources.
- Issues relating to practice when working with those who deliberately self-harm should be discussed in clinical supervision sessions.
- Clinicians should endeavour to support each other whilst working within the clinical environment.
- Clinicians should access and network with other groups and agencies involved in the care of those who self-injure.
- Clinicians should assist in the development of change and acceptance in relation to people who self-injure.

Clinical considerations

1. Strategies aimed at management of self-harm within forensic mental health care should be tailored to the individual.
2. Continuous observation may prove counterproductive.
3. Thorough assessment is of paramount importance, including a detailed history of self-harm and incidents of aggression if appropriate.
4. Clear guidelines for practice are a fundamental requirement for effective care delivery.

Conclusion

Self-harm may always remain a mystery to some clinicians, but this should not be a barrier to offering effective care. Education, support and supervision for practitioners should be made available. Misconceptions must be challenged and the need to care reinforced.

Self-harm is not a reason for incarceration within forensic mental health services. It may, nevertheless, be one aspect of an individual's presentation, which warrants attention. In such circumstances it is crucial that therapeutic aims are tailored to the individual's needs, are realistic and achievable. Progress should not be measured against the number or severity of incidents of self-harm, as the issues are more complex. Effective care requires sensitivity and understanding. These approaches can be enhanced through collaboration between survivor groups, user-led organisations and mental health care professionals.

Consideration of an issue such as self-harm is of limited worth if it is not translated into practice, a process in which, as mental health care workers, we all have a shared responsibility. Service provision continues to develop but good practice needs to be disseminated in order to provide a consistent, comprehensive and effective service to those who may require it.

References

Allen, C. (1995) Helping with deliberate self-harm: some practical guidelines. *Journal of Mental Health*, 4, pp. 243–50.

Allen, S. (1997) An Examination of the Ethnicity of Females who Self-Harm Within the Forensic Mental Health Service. Unpublished thesis, Reaside Clinic, Birmingham.

Anderson, M. (1997) Nurses' attitudes toward suicidal behaviour – a comparative study of community mental health nurses and nurses working in an Accident and Emergency Department. *Journal of Advanced Nursing*, 25, pp. 1283–91.

Arnold, L. (1995) *Women and Self-Injury: A Survey of 76 Women*. Bristol Crisis Service for Women, Bristol.

Arnold, L. (1997) *Working With People Who Self-Injure – A Training Pack*. Bristol Crisis Service for Women, Bristol.

Arnold, L. and Magill, A. (1996) *Working With Self-Injury: A Practical Guide*. The Basement Project, Abergavenny.

Arnold, L. and Magill, A. (1998) *The Self-Harm Help Book*. The Basement Project, Abergavenny.

Babiker, G. and Arnold, L. (1997) *The Language of Injury: Comprehending Self-Mutilation*. The British Psychological Society, Leicester.

Bailey, S. (1994) Critical care nurses' and doctors' attitudes to parasuicide patients. *Australian Journal of Advanced Nursing*, 11 (3), pp. 11–17.

Barnes, R. (1982) Women and self-injury. *International Journal of Women's Studies*, 8 (5), pp. 465–74.

Barstow, D. (1995) Self-injury and self-mutilation – nursing approaches. *Journal of Psychosocial Nursing*, 33 (2), pp. 19–22.

Beasley, S. (1999) Aspects of Deliberate Self-Harm in a Regional Secure Unit: A Three Part Study. Unpublished thesis, Reaside Clinic, Birmingham.

Bunclark, J. and Adcock, C. (1996) Signs of self-harm. *Practice Nurse*, June, pp. 699–704.

Burnham, R.C. (1969) Symposium on Impulsive Self-Mutilation: Discussion. *British Journal of Medical Psychology*, 42, pp. 223–9.

Burrow, S. (1992) The deliberate self-harming behaviour of patients within a British special hospital, *Journal of Advanced Nursing*, 17, 138–48.

Burrow, S. (1994) Nursing management of self-mutilation. *British Journal of Nursing*, 3 (8), pp. 382–6.

Casale, S. (1989) *Women Inside*. Civil Liberties Trust, London.

Clarke, L. and Whittaker, M. (1998) Self-mutilation: culture, contexts and nursing responses. *Journal of Clinical Nursing*, 7 (2), pp. 129–37.

Department of Health (1999a) Code of Practice – Mental Health Health Act 1983. DoH, London.

Department of Health (1999b) Practice Guidance: Safe and Supportive Observation of Patients at Risk. Standing Nursing and Midwifery Advisory Committee. DoH, London.

Dollard, J., Doob, L., Miller, N., Mowrer, O. H. and Sears, R.R. (1939) *Frustration and Aggression*. Yale University Press, New Haven, CT. Cited in Favazza (1996).

Eliade, M. (1975) *Rites and Symbols of Initiation*. Harper and Row, New York.

Favazza, A.R. (1989) Why patients mutilate themselves. *Hospital and Community Psychiatry*, 40 (2), pp. 137–45.

Favazza, A.R. (1996) *Bodies Under Siege: Self-Mutilation and Body Modification in Culture and Psychiatry*, 2nd edn. The Johns Hopkins University Press, London.

Favazza, A.R. and Conterio, K. (1988) The plight of chronic self-mutilators. *Community Mental Health Journal*, 24 (1), pp. 22–30.

Favazza, A.R. and Conterio, K. (1989) Female habitual self-mutilators. *Acta Psychiatry Scandinavica*, 79, pp. 283–9.

Favazza, A.R. and Simeon, D. (1995) Self-mutilation. In E. Hollander and D. Stein (eds), *Impulsivity and Aggression*. John Wiley and Sons, Chichester, pp. 185–200.

Faye, P. (1995) Addictive characteristics of the behaviour of self-mutilation. *Journal of Psychological Nursing*, 33 (6), pp. 36–9.

Fraser, K. and Gallop, R. (1993) Nurses' confirming/disconfirming responses to patients diagnosed with borderline personality disorder. *Archives of Psychiatric Nursing*, 7 (6), pp. 336–41.

Gallop, R., Lancee, W. and Shugar, G. (1993) Residents' and nurses' perceptions of difficult to treat short-stay patients. *Hospital and Community Psychiatry*, 44 (4), pp. 352–7.

Gardener, A.R. and Gardener, A.J. (1975) Self-mutilation, obsessionality and narcissism. *British Journal of Psychiatry*, 127, 127–32.

Garner, R. and Butler, G. (1994) Learning from acts of deliberate self-harm. A study of self-inflicted injury in a secure unit. *Psychiatric Care*, (Nov–Dec), pp. 197–201.

Garner, R., Butler, G. and Hutchings, D. (1996) A study of the relationship between the patterns of planned activity and incidents of self-harm within a regional secure unit. *British Journal of Occupational Therapy*, 59 (4), 156–60.

Ghodse, A.H., Ghaffari, K., Bhat, A.V., Gelea, A. and Qureshi, Y.H. (1986) Attitudes of health care professionals towards patients who take overdoses. *International Journal of Social Psychiatry*, 32 (4), 58–63.

Gibbs, A. (1990) Aspects of communication with people who have attempted suicide. *Journal of*

Advanced Nursing, 15, 1245–9.

Hardie, T.J. (1998) Self-harm shows diurnal variation. *Criminal Behaviour and Mental Health*, 8, 17–18.

Harrison, D. (1995) Vicious circles – an exploration of women and self-harm in society. GPMH Publications, London.

Hawton, K. and Catalan, J. (1987) *Attempted Suicide: A Practical Guide to its Nature and Management*, 2nd edn. Oxford University Press, Oxford.

Hawton, K. (1990) Self-cutting: can it be prevented? In K. Hawton and P. Cowen, *Dilemmas and Difficulties in the Management of Psychiatric Patients*. Oxford Medical Publications, Oxford, pp. 91–103.

Hawton, K., Fagg, J., Simkin, S., Bale, E., and Bond, A. (1997) Trends in deliberate self-harm in Oxford, 1985–1995. *British Journal of Psychiatry*, 171, 556–60.

Hemkendries, M. (1992) Increase in self-injuries on an inpatient psychiatric unit during evening hours. *Hospital and Community Psychiatry*, 43 (4), 394–5.

Hemmings, A. (1997) Calls for help. *Health Service Journal*, 12 June, pp. 34–5.

Hillbrand, M. (1992) Self-directed and other directed aggressive behaviour in a forensic sample. *Suicide and Life Threatening Behaviour*, 22 (3), pp. 333–40.

Hillis, G. and McClelland, N. (1998) Cycle of alienation. *Nursing Times*, 30 September, 94 (39), pp. 29–30.

Hogg, C.(1996) Two-edged sword of publicity. *Nursing Times*, 10 July, 92 (28), p. 16.

Inch, H., Rowlands, P. and Soliman, A. (1995) Deliberate self-harm in a young offenders' institution. *Journal of Forensic Psychiatry*, 6 (1), 161–71.

Johnstone, L. (1997) Why do Medical Explanations of Self-Harm do More Harm Than Good? From the Conference Proceedings 'Managing Self-Harm: What? Why? How?' Henderson Hospital, Surrey.

Kahan, J. and Pattison, M. (1984) Proposal for a distinctive diagnosis: the deliberate self-harm syndrome. *Suicide and Life Threatening Behaviour*, 14, pp. 17–35.

Kapur, N., House, A., Creed, F., Feldman, E., Friedman, T. and Guthrie, E. (1999) Hospital management of deliberate self-harm: towards quality and consistency. *Mental Health Care*, 1 (5), pp. 170–3.

Konicki, P.E. and Schultz, S.C. (1989) Rationale for clinical trials of opiate antagonists in treating patients with personality disorders and self-injurious behaviour. *Psychopharmacology Bulletin*, 25 (4), pp. 556–63.

Liebling, A. (1992) *Suicides in Prison*. Routledge Books, London.

Liebling, A. (1995) Vulnerability and prison suicide. *British Journal of Criminology*, 35 (2), pp. 173–85.

Loughrey, L., Jackson, J., Molla, P. and Wobbleton, J. (1997) Patient self-mutilation: when nursing becomes a nightmare. *Journal of Psychosocial Nursing*, 35 (4), pp. 30–4.

McGaughey, J. and Harrison, S. (1995) Suicide and parasuicide: a selected review of the literature. *Journal of Psychiatric and Mental Health Nursing*, 2, 199–206.

McLaughlin, C. (1994) Casualty nurses' attitudes to attempted suicide. *Journal of Advanced Nursing*, 20, pp. 1111–18.

Melville, A. and House, A. (1998) Deliberate self-harm. *Health Service Journal*, 10 December, pp. 34–5.

Mental Health Foundation (1997) *Suicide and Deliberate Self-Harm – The Fundamental Facts.* MHF Briefing No.1. MHF, London.

Merrill, J. and Owens, J. (1988) Self-poisoning among four immigrant groups. *Acta Psychiatry Scandinavica*, 77, 77–80.

Miller, D. (1994) *Women Who Hurt Themselves: A Book of Hope and Understanding.* Basic Books, New York.

Morse, J.M. and Mitcham, C. (1997) Compathy: the contagion of physical distress. *Journal of Advanced Nursing*, 26, 649–57.

Pattison, E. and Kahan, J. (1983) The deliberate self-harm syndrome. *American Journal of Psychiatry*, 140 (7), pp. 867–72.

Pembroke, L. (1991) Surviving psychiatry. *Nursing Times*, 87 (49), 30–2.

Pembroke, L. (1994) *Self-Harm: Perspectives from Personal Experience*. Survivors Speak Out, London (ISBN 1 898002 02 9).

Pembroke, L. (1998) Self-harm: a personal story. *Mental Health Practice*, 2 (2), pp. 20–4.

Powell, G. and Wyatt, G.E. (1988) *Lasting Effects of Child Sexual Abuse*. Sage Publications, London.

Romans, S., Martin, J., Anderson, J., Herbison, G. and Mullen, P. (1995) Sexual abuse in childhood and deliberate self-harm. *American Journal of Psychiatry*, 152 (9), pp. 1336–42.

Rosenthal, R.J., Rinzler, C., Walsh, R. and Klausner, E. (1972) Wrist-cutting syndrome: the meaning of a gesture. *American Journal of Psychiatry*, 128, 11.

Ross, R.R. and McKay, H.B. (1979) *Self-Mutilation*. Lexington Books, London.

Russ, M.J. (1992) Self-injurious behaviour in patients with borderline personality disorder: biological perspectives. *Journal of Personality Disorders*, 6 (1), pp. 64–81.

Sakinofsky, I. and Roberts, R.S. (1990) Why parasuicides repeat despite problem resolution. *British Journal of Psychiatry*, 156, 399–405.

Shugar, G. and Rehaluk, R. (1990) Continuous observation for psychiatric inpatients: a critical evaluation. *Comprehensive Psychiatry*, 30 (1), pp. 48–55.

Simpson, M. A. (1975) Symposium – Self-Injury: The Phenomenology of Self-Mutilation in a General Hospital Setting. *Canadian Psychiatric Association Journal*, 20 (6), 429–34.

Simpson, A. and Ng, M. (1992) Deliberate self-harm in Filipino immigrants in Hong Kong. *International Journal of Psychology in the Orient*, 35 (2), pp. 117–20.

Soni Raleigh, V. and Balarajan, R. (1992) Suicide and self-burning among Indians and West Indians in England and Wales. *British Journal of Psychiatry*, 161, pp. 365–8.

Stengal, E. (1970) *Suicide and Attempted Suicide*, 2nd edn. Penguin Books, Harmondsworth.

Swinton, M. and Hopkins, R. (1996) Violence and self-injury. *Journal of Forensic Psychiatry*, 7, 563–9.

Taiminen, T.J., Kallio-Soukainen, K., Nakso-Koivisto, H., Kaljonen, A. and Helenius, H. (1998) Contagion of deliberate self-harm amongst adolescent inpatients. *American Academy of Child and Adolescent Psychiatry*, 37 (2), pp. 211–17.

Tantum, D. and Whitaker, J. (1992) Personality disorder and self-wounding. *British Journal of Psychiatry*, 161, pp. 451–64.

Thornton, D. (1990) Depression, self-injury and attempted suicide amongst the YOI population. In Proceedings of the Prison Psychologists Conference. Division of Psychological Services Report Series I: 34, pp. 47–55.

Van der Kolk, B.A., Perry, C. and Hermen, J. (1991) Childhood origins of self-destructive behaviour. *American Journal of Psychiatry*, 148, p. 12.

Virkkunen, M. (1976) Self-mutilation and anti-social personality disorder. *Acta Psychiatry Scandinavica*, 54, 347–52.

Walsh, B.W. and Rosen, P.M. (1988) *Self-Mutilation: Theory, Research and Treatment*. The Guilford Press, New York.

Weissman, M.M. (1975) Wrist cutting: relationship between clinical observations and epidemiological findings. *Archives of General Psychiatry*, 32 (September), pp. 1166–71.

Winkler, G. (1992) Assessing and responding to suicidal jail inmates. *Community Mental Health Journal*, 28 (4), pp. 317–26.

White, J., Leggett, J. and Beech, A. (1999) The incidence of self-harming behaviour in the male population of a medium secure psychiatric hospital. *Journal of Forensic Psychiatry*, 10 (1), 59–68.

Wilkins, J. and Coid, J. (1991) Self-mutilation in female remanded prisoners: an indicator of severe psychopathology. *Criminal Behaviour and Mental Health*, 1, pp. 247–67.

Williams, R. and Morgan, G. for the National Health Service Advisory Committee (1994) *Suicide Prevention: The Challenge Confronted – Thematic Review*.

Winchel, R. and Stanley, M. (1991) Self-injurious behaviour: a review of the behaviour and biology of self-mutilation. *American Journal of Psychiatry*, 148 (3), pp. 306–17.

6 Legal aspects

Martin Humphreys, Emmanuel Oppong-Gyapong and Dave Mason

Historically, statutory mental health legislation in the United Kingdom, particularly from the second half of the eighteenth century onwards, has been designed to be operated mainly by medical practitioners and defined by statute and common law (Bluglass, 1983). Prior to that it had been intended primarily to provide measures for the social control of mentally disordered people. With the growth of psychiatry came an increase in understanding of disorders of the mind and their treatment. This, together with the so-called 'open door' model of care and the more prominent place given to human rights and civil liberties in society as a whole, and the acknowledgement that mental disorder had much in common with physical ill health, was reflected in new legislation introduced in the United Kingdom in the late 1950s, which presumed the right to treatment on a voluntary basis. Previously the emphasis has been upon involuntary measures, compulsory admission to hospital and treatment of patients in large institutions. With time, matters concerned with the civil rights of the mentally disordered, not only in relation to voluntary access to services, but also the capacity to exercise their own will and judgement and make decisions, came under increasing scrutiny (Gostin, 1975, 1977). After a prolonged and careful review process and wide consultation, the Mental Health Act 1983 became law.

The nurse's statutory duties and responsibilities

The statutory duties of mental health care nurses are relatively well circumscribed. This is perhaps curious given the fact that nurses are members of the single professional group who have the most consistent, frequent and prolonged direct contact with patients both in hospital and community settings. There are, nevertheless, two important areas, both of which reflect the vital nature of that relationship, one of which involves the immediate and uncensored removal of a patient's liberty and the other which is very much concerned with the nurse's central role in patient care and their knowledge and understanding of the individual and their treatment needs.

Nurses' holding powers

The Mental Health Act 1983 made a significant change from previous legislation in giving registered nurses the power to detain, for up to six hours, an informal patient already in hospital. It makes provision for this where it becomes evident that an application should be made for admission for assessment or treatment, but there is insufficient time to pursue any alternative course of action. Section 5(4) of the Act states that:

> If, in the case of a patient who is receiving treatment for mental disorder as an in-patient in a hospital, it appears to a nurse that the prescribed class:
>
> (a) that the patient is suffering from mental disorder to such a degree that it is necessary for his health or safety or the protection of others for him to be immediately restrained from leaving the hospital; and
>
> (b) that is not practicable to secure the immediate attendance of a practitioner for the purpose of furnishing a report under subsection (2) above,
>
> the nurse may record that fact in writing; and in that event the patient may be detained in the hospital for a period of six hours from the time when that fact is so recorded or until the earlier arrival at the place where the patient is detained of a practitioner having power to furnish a report under that subsection.

According to the Code of Practice to the Act, the six-hour period of holding commences when the written record is made and this must be delivered to the hospital managers either by the nurse concerned or someone authorised by them to do so.

There is broadly similar provision for nurses' holding powers in the Mental Health (Scotland) Act 1984, which differs only in the fact that it allows for a maximum of two hours' detention. Nurses' holding powers are important. They place the responsibility for the identification of mental disorder and its degree of severity, as well as the likely outcome if the individual is allowed to leave, on a single clinician. The period of detention is limited and intended to allow for the attendance of a medical practitioner and, where appropriate, the pursuit of an application or recommendation for a further period of compulsory care. This provision under the 1983 Act was new and arose out of the need to provide a formal means for nurses to hold patients when no doctor was available to see them. The use of nurses' holding power varies, both geographically (Pourgourides *et al.*, 1992; Mason and Turner, 1994) and in the same place over time (Salib, 1998). They are used for a variety of reasons (Pym *et al.*, 1999), not least due to concerns over the potential for adverse events to occur if patients are at liberty (Ashmore, 1992).

Given that nurses' holding powers allow for the removal of an individual's right to freedom, there has been considerable concern expressed over the apparent lack of knowledge of them, particularly among those who one might expect to have the most clear and up-to-date understanding, and be in a position to use them (Ashmore, 1992). Despite those concerns, like their medical counterparts whose knowledge may be equally limited (Bhatti *et al.*, 1999a), nurses do seem to make broadly appropriate decisions in relation to holding powers (Pym *et al.*, 1999). In practice, whether nurses' holding powers are used depends upon a wide variety of different factors. They can be associated particularly with episodes of hostility and aggression towards others, but also concerns over the potential for self-harm. In reality, the situation may depend upon the ability to manage and control a difficult, or potentially difficult situation, and persuade a disturbed or hostile patient to stay voluntarily and await the arrival of a doctor.

Consent to treatment

Perhaps the single most important statutory role fulfilled by the nurse is that which relates to the provision for consent to treatment. In relation to both treatment that requires consent and a second opinion (surgery for the destruction of brain tissue or function or any other form of specified treatment), or that requiring consent or a second opinion (essentially the administration of medication beyond three months where the patient is either unwilling or unable to consent), the appointed second opinion doctor is required by law to consult with certain others who are involved in the patient's treatment, one of whom must be a nurse. This is therefore a pivotal role. The nurse is someone with knowledge of treatment and clinical expertise, an understanding of the patient and their circumstances and wider needs, who is able to comment on the patient's personal and family situation from a position of authority, but also a close therapeutic relationship. They can offer a professional view, but one independent of the responsible medical officer or physician in charge of the case. They can act as facilitator and advocate. This is clearly then an important function and responsibility and one that should not be undertaken lightly. The content and outcome of consultation with second opinion doctors may have a profound and prolonged effect on the future of the therapeutic relationship with the patient and the outcome of their treatment.

Changing health policy and its effect on care provision

As the role of the nurse became extended to encompass an increasingly holistic perception of the patient, embracing a widening body of knowledge, this in turn gave rise to increasingly innovative strategies for care in the move away from a traditional illness focus.

During the 1980s the Conservative government in the United Kingdom announced plans to scale down the in-patient population of many of the country's psychiatric hospitals, thereby prioritising the reintegration of people with enduring mental health problems, into their own communities. The rationale offered by the government for this radical shift in health care provision was in order to counteract what had been broadly studied and accepted as the concept of institutionalisation.

Goffman (1961) has suggested that hospitals became dumping grounds, which in turn stigmatised, alienated and demoralised patients. The advent of community care offered an opportunity to further balance power within the nurse/patient relationship, with the patient afforded greater involvement in the way in which care was to be planned. In addition, advances in drug therapies available offered the benefit of reducing the range of side-effects which had traditionally hampered compliance. This offered the possibility of enhancing quality of life, as demonstrated by Franz *et al.* (1997) in their comparison of the effects of atypical neuroleptic medication vs. conventional neuroleptics on the subjective quality of life in patients suffering from schizophrenia.

Hart (1999), however, questions the government's therapeutic motive in the institution of community care, arguing that health care is poorly planned and economically driven. She is not alone in her condemnation of community care. The issue of caring for the mentally ill in the community has remained a source of great public anxiety as a result of numerous incidents where patients have committed serious criminal offences. Most significant of these incidents in terms of its implications for the future of mental health care policy was the murder in 1992 of Jonathan Zito by Christopher Clunis, who, at the time of the offence, had a history of psychiatric care which dated back six years, although the mental health services responsible for his aftercare had been unable to maintain contact with him. Since the publication of the Report of the Committee of Inquiry into the care and treatment of Christopher Clunis (Ritchie, 1994), concern has continued to grow amid the subsequent inquiries into the deaths of people at the hands of mentally ill people in the community, and the increased media attention which such incidents have attracted. Many of the inquiries have shown significant shortcomings in the way in which community care has been administered.

In 1991, the Care Programme Approach was introduced and outlined a statutory requirement that health authorities and social services departments should devise and implement care packages for all patients in contact with specialist mental health services. Despite this, however, Zito (1998) reported that the care programme approach had not been implemented in a number of health authorities inspected by the Department of Health in 1995.

Other criticisms of community care have revolved around nursing staff failing to engage with patients and to adequately provide follow-up care. Hart (1999) criticises the lack of defined national framework for the implementation of community care in addition to the poor availability of specialist training for nurses working in the community setting (Saggers and McClelland, 1999).

Birmingham (1999), when comparing the progress of community care in Britain with similar programmes of health care reform which were undertaken earlier in America, suggests that evidence is now emerging that indicates that the closure of psychiatric hospitals coupled with an under-resourced community care system may result in prisons replacing hospitals as the main provider of institutional care for the mentally ill, as has occurred in America. The varying views as to why community care has failed to achieve its full potential have compounded an issue which has given rise to a regression in the public perception of people who suffer from mental illness to one which presumes a predisposition to violent behaviour or even homicidal potential.

Therefore, the difficulty for successive governments has been in the provision of adequate supervision and quality of care for the mentally ill in the community, whilst reassuring an anxious public, in a manner which does not represent a significant economic burden.

The government sought to address this through the introduction of the Mental Health (Patients in the Community) Act 1995. The purpose of the 1995 Act was to offer increased security through supervision whilst striving to prevent the problem of the 'revolving door patient', where frequent periods of involuntary in-patient care during periods of acute illness, followed by discharge as a result of successful treatment are eventually followed by readmission as a consequence of refusal to comply with aftercare arrangements.

Under the 1995 Act, 'supervised discharge', a revision and extension of the guardianship aspect of the Mental Health Act 1983, was viewed as a means to ensure improved rates of compliance with aftercare as an adjunct to legislative mechanisms already in place, such as the Care Programme Approach and Section 117 of the Mental Health Act 1983. Supervised discharge effectively strengthened powers of community teams through the prescription of conditions to which the patient must agree prior to discharge whilst acknowledging that failure to comply may cause the team responsible to enact their right under the act to 'take and convey' them to a place where the issue of non-compliance may be addressed and where necessary, assessment for compulsory admission may be facilitated. The power to take and convey a community based patient 'to a place where they are required to reside or attend for medical treatment, occupation, education or training' (Department of Health, 1995), has presented significant challenges to both nurses and those in their care. This has been largely due to the anxiety this has provoked in both camps. Repper *et al.* (1994) suggest that this authority represents a power of arrest and that its 'principle of compulsion will further undermine the partnership philosophy of patient involvement in determining their care plans'.

This, according to Coyne (1999), represents a direct conflict between the roles of carer and controller and between legislation and the concept of empowerment. He therefore concludes that this would result in patients avoiding contact with mental health services through fear of compulsory treatment. Other critics of the Act, Fulop (1995) for example, have complained that its powers are insufficient to address the issue of non-compliance with medication. Slinger (1997) highlights this when she suggests that, despite the detail included in an aftercare plan and the potential for it to produce a successful treatment outcome, health care professionals remain powerless if the symptom-free (and therefore ineligible for compulsory admission) patient chooses not to participate.

The 1995 Act stipulates that, even if the power to take and convey is enacted, 'the patient cannot then be required to accept treatment' (Department of Health, 1995) and that 'the power should only be used if the supervisor is satisfied that the act of removal will lead to the patient's co-operation with services' (Department of Health, 1995). Despite this rationale, the Act also stipulates that 'Unreasonable force must never be used when conveying a patient, and neither should the power (or the threat of using it) be used to coerce a patient into accepting medication or treatment' (Department of Health, 1995). Many professionals and user groups concerned about the implications for future mental health practice have drawn attention to the paradoxical nature of this critical aspect of the legislation.

In late 1998 the former Health Secretary, Frank Dobson, announced his plans for a 'third way' for mental health services in which he condemned community care as having been a 'failure' whilst unveiling a strategy that would strengthen the concept through increased resources and the widespread implementation of measures such as Assertive Outreach teams.

Previous plans to implement Community Treatment Orders in 1993 (then termed Community Supervision Orders), which had been proposed by the Royal College of Psychiatrists, were rejected by the Health Select Committee, who reviewed the evidence describing them as 'fundamentally flawed' (Linehan, 1993).

Sandford (1993) advocated a more detailed examination of the problems which had brought about calls for community supervision orders, observing that:

> Proposals were founded on little more than compelling patients to take neuroleptic medication but failed to consider the reasons why patients do not comply with treatment packages which rely on this approach. Reliance upon neuroleptic drugs has deflected attention away from more creative ways of dealing with illness. (Sandford, 1993, pp. 22–3)

Bluglass (1993) discussing the prospect of nurses administering intramuscular medication without consent in the patient's home describes this potential scenario as 'unacceptable and unethical'.

Despite the swell of condemnation and rejection of earlier proposals to implement community treatment orders, little has changed that would indicate acceptance of such a strategy for care today. Indeed, widespread rejection of the concept has been the result of this aspect of the 'third way' for mental health, with many user groups such as MIND warning that compulsory treatment would drive users away from services. Despite continued concern from all areas of the mental health profession it would appear that the, no doubt, imminent arrival of compulsory community treatment will represent the ultimate test of the nurse/patient relationship.

Possible future developments

Currently there is consideration being given to sweeping reform and changes in mental health legislation across most of the United Kingdom. It seems unlikely at this early stage in the process that this will have any major effect on the statutory duties and responsibilities of psychiatric nurses, but it may have implications for service delivery, the spectrum of disorder seen, particularly among detained patients, as well as changes in health care facilities, especially in terms of secure provision. It is proposed that the term 'psychopathic disorder' be removed from the 1983 Act for England and Wales. It may be replaced by the more clinically orientated 'personality disorder', but this may do little to clarify the legal or therapeutic dilemmas associated with patients with related problems and the statutory legal category.

An area in which nursing practice and professional and ethical standards may be challenged in the future is that related to the potential for the introduction of compulsory community treatment orders. Although reservations have been expressed among various groups of mental health care professionals, there are those who are very much in favour of such provision, despite the potential for infringement of civil rights (Bhatti *et al.*, 1999b). It is likely that if community treatment orders are incorporated into new mental health legislation, they will be used, and that in those circumstances community staff from all disciplines, particularly nurses, may have a lead role to play, both at the stage of initiating the order and implementing it once in place. This could include the use of measures to ensure compulsory treatment of patients in their own homes. The ethical and moral dilemmas associated with this form of compulsion are self-evident. The practicalities of this form of intervention remain unaddressed. It is possible, given what has transpired in the past, that where legislative measures are unpopular or deemed impracticable or unhelpful by mental health care professionals, they will remain unused (Bhatti *et al.*, 1999b).

References

Ashmore, R. (1992) The use of Section 5 (4) to detain patients. *Nursing Times*, 87 (4), pp. 58–9.

Bhatti, V., Kenney Herbert, J.P., Cope R.V. and Humphreys, M.S. (1999a) Knowledge of current mental health legislation among medical practitioners approved under Section 12 (2) of the Mental Health Act 1983 in the West Midlands. *Health Trends*, 4, pp. 106–8.

Bhatti, V., Kenney Herbert, J.P., Cope R.V. and Humphreys, M.S. (1999b) The Mental Health Act 1983. Views of section 12 (2) approved doctors on selected areas of current legislation. *Psychiatric Bulletin*, 23, pp. 534–6.

Birmingham, L. (1999) Between prison and community: the revolving door patient of the nineties. *British Journal of Psychiatry*, 174, pp. 378–9.

Bluglass, R. (1993) The case for supervision. *Nursing Times*, 10 February, 89 (6).

Coyne, A. (1999) Supervised discharge: a time for debate. *Mental Health Practice* 2 (8).

Department of Health and Welsh Office (1999) Code of Practice: Mental Health Act 1983. Department of Health, London.

Franz, M., Lis, S., Pluddermann, K. and Gallhofer, B. (1997) Conventional versus atypical neuroleptics: subjective quality of life in schizophrenic patients. *British Journal of Psychiatry*, 170, pp. 422–5.

Fulop, N. (1995) Supervised discharge: lessons from the U.S. experience. *Mental Health Nursing*, 15 (3), pp. 16–20.

Goffman, E. (1961). *Asylums – Essays on the Social Situation of Mental Patients and Other Inmates*. Pelican, Middlesex.

Gostin, L. (1975) A human condition I. National Association of Mental Health: London.

Gostin, L. (1977) A human condition II. National Association of Mental Health: London.

Hart, C. (1999) Keeping teams together. *Nursing Times*, 15 September, 95 (37), pp. 48–9.

Linehan, T. (1993) Taking control. *Nursing Times*, 28 July, 89 (30) p. 19.

Mason, P. and Turner, R. (1994) Audit of the use of doctors' holding power under Section 5 (2) of the Mental Health Act 1983. *Health Trends*, 26, pp. 44–6.

Pourgourides, C., Prasher, V.P. and Oyebode, F. (1992) Use of Section 5 (2) in clinical practice. *Psychiatric Bulletin*, 16, pp. 14–16.

Pym, N., Bell, C. and Salib, E. (1999) A review of 100 applications of Section 5 (4) of the Mental Health Act 1983. *Nursing Standard*, 13, pp. 37–40.

Repper, J., Forde, R. and Cooke, A. (1994) How can nurses build trusting relationships with people who have severe and long term mental health problems? Experiences of case managers and their clients. *Journal of Advanced Nursing*, 19, pp. 1096–104.

Ritchie, J.H. (Chairman), Dick, D. and Lingham, R. (1994) *Report of the Inquiry into the Care and Treatment of Christopher Clunis*. HMSO, London.

Saggers, J. and McClelland, N. (1999) How informed are community psychiatric nurses of their role in the implementation of supervised discharge? *Medicine, Science and the Law*, 39, 313–18.

Salib, E. (1998) Audit of the use of nurses' holding power under section 5 (4) of the Mental Health Act 1984. *Medicine Science and the Law*, 38, 227–32.

Sandford, T. (1993) Supervision Orders: where next? *Nursing Standard*, 4 August, 7 (46), pp. 22–3.

Slinger, P. (1997) Supervised aftercare for clients with mental health problems. *Nursing Times*, 22 October, 93 (43), pp. 50–1.

Zito, J. (1998) Lessons from the outside. *Nursing Times*, 28 January, 94 (4), 34–5.

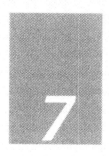

Education, and training

Norman McClelland and Joe Cutler

The Forensic Mental Health nursing literature is expanding to the degree that many works are re-examining what some consider to be a baseline knowledge, and standardised set of practical skills, necessary for forensic nursing practice. Collins (2000) has provided an excellent overview of procedures in secure settings, some of which relate to the practitioner new to the role of forensic psychiatric nursing. This knowledge and repertoire of baseline skills is necessary for practice in a range of healthcare settings, which are deemed as secure, or related to forensic practice. Kettles and Robinson (2000) relate a survey conducted by themselves (Kettles and Robinson 1998) of ten secure units in Scotland and England. This study was made to address issues of forensic nursing, amongst them what sort of training was required. They write of nurses in these units indicating that they would like more training in areas related to 'The Prison Service', the Criminal Procedures Act, dangerousness and manipulative behaviours (Kettles and Robinson, 2000, p. 34).

A range of training also must complement any form of education provision within an organisation such as a forensic secure hospital. Nurses and other professionals must be able to function adequately, and require a broad awareness of specific procedures to enable them to do so. Hence many secure units have developed an in-house programme of training, some of which incorporates an academic component related to areas such as self-harm, risk assessment and the law as it relates to the Mental Health Act 1983 (Home Office, 1983).

It is anticipated that the provision of in-house training and development programmes will help develop staff, as well as promote organisational philosophies, attitudes, skills and practices which have been devised to meet service needs. Secure services can be very sophisticated in terms of the way they deliver care, and it is to be expected that the modern secure environment will provide knowledge and develop skills above the minimum statutory requirement. It is perhaps expected that service needs analysis and staff development needs would promote a diverse programme of workshops and courses, designed to create a health care workforce competent at a predetermined level.

Induction and preceptorship

Storey and Dale (1999) in their recent Scope document state that:

> Induction of staff into a new post or a new role should be seen as an investment. The Inductee should be confident that they are familiar with policies, protocols and working practices as soon as possible on commencement in the job. (Storey and Dale, 1999, p. 100)

The induction into a secure environment should cover the range of varied and unique organisational issues. This will invariably include an introduction to the organisational structure, as well as key personnel within the organisation and the range of service provision. The roles and responsibilities of the new member of staff should be outlined as well as key security issues, policies and protocols. These will relate to health and safety and welfare issues, as well as those specific to the patient group. It is likely that areas to be addressed will include treatment, relationships and boundaries, ethical and legal issues, cultural awareness, multiprofessional working and managing challenging behaviours.

At Reaside Clinic in Birmingham, the induction programme for new clinical staff is a three-day theory based programme, has multidisciplinary input and is designed for a multidisciplinary audience. Students from each of the clinical professions undertake the induction also. It is believed to be very important to have a common induction for all staff, this serves the purpose of bridging barriers between professions as well as improving understanding of how a range of staff work and function within the service.

The induction programme is co-ordinated by a staff development officer and includes the following:

- **Day One**
1. An introduction to the Trust and Reaside Clinic. Philosophy, general policy, charter of rights and organisational structure of the Trust.
2. A tour of the clinic and training in the use of passes, alarms, and keys.
3. A demographic overview of residents including diagnosis/index offence /ethnicity race and culture.
4. Multidisciplinary working – including the function of clinical teams.
- **Day Two**
1. Security – including professional boundaries and confidentiality.
2. Policies and procedures – including equal opportunities, harassment, staff support systems and Trust and clinic policies.
3. The role of the occupational therapist.
4. Predispositional factors associated with violence and an introduction to risk assessment.
- **Day Three**
1. Self-harming behaviour.
2. Mental Health Act (emphasis on part III).
3. The role of the psychologist.
4. Attendance at the weekly clinic-wide clinical presentation.
5. Health and safety – including infection control/waste disposal/lifting and handling/HIV awareness.
6. The role of the forensic mental health nurse.

This programme is delivered by a range of staff that are employed within the clinic, drawn from a range of disciplines. There is a formal evaluation of the students' perception of the programme, as well as a gradual introduction to moving around the clinic with passes, keys and alarms.

Nursing staff go through a further four-week unit based induction within the clinical area. Here they are assigned a supervisor whose role it is to further familiarise the inductee with the organisation and unit philosophy. The inductee and supervisor complete a competency checklist during this period, and this is then retained on an employee's personal file.

Following induction, a newly qualified member of nursing staff will be assigned a preceptor, to assist development of the staff member over a four- to six-month period, dependent upon specific learning needs. Prior to commencing the preceptorship process, the preceptor and preceptee attend a half-day workshop to aid understanding of the process, and to further examine competencies associated with the role. They will further examine how to negotiate learning contracts and targets to achieve in a designated period. Nursing assistants or experienced nursing staff new to the clinic will, following induction, be assigned a mentor, to assist them in adapting to the new role and the organisation.

Clinical supervision

The necessity for all nursing staff to receive clinical supervision is acknowledged by the UKCC in its positional statement on clinical supervision for nursing and health visiting (1995). This document relates how 'clinical supervision supports practice, enabling practitioners to maintain and promote standards of care' (UKCC, 1995). Although clinical supervision is not at present a statutory requirement, the UKCC (1995) recognise that 'the potential impact on care and professional development is sufficient to merit investment in clinical supervision. It also makes a significant contribution to clinical risk management while maintaining staff morale and aiding recruitment' (UKCC, 1995).

Addo (2000) writes of the complexity of working with mentally disordered offenders, and of how this reflects the complexity of the working environment as well as the complication of legal constraints on care management and the patient's position. The close working relationship forensic mental health nurses have with other professionals requires that clinical supervision, if employed, can assist the nurse in developing a range of skills.

Clinical supervision at Reaside Clinic is seen as an integral part of the development of the nurse. To this end a model of clinical supervision has been adapted and modified to suit the specific requirements of nursing in a secure environment. The model used is an adaptation of Proctor's (1988) three-function interactive model. The three functions, 'formative, restorative and normative', are, according to Proctor, processes that occur within clinical supervision. The inclusion of a 'contract' of supervision between supervisor and supervisee assists in the setting of boundaries for the process and helps identify specific elements of professional practice to be addressed in the sessions. The supervisee chooses a supervisor (within certain guidelines) and is also responsible for keeping all the notes and copies of the contract. The supervision usually takes place on a monthly basis, but there is the facility for the supervision to be 'live' if required, particularly following unusual or traumatic experiences within the supervisee's daily practice. The Forensic Mental Health Nurse's role has within it many ambiguities, not least the dual role of providing the most appropriate level of security whilst maintaining a therapeutic rapport with patients. The exposure to, encouragement and promotion of, a model of clinical supervision can significantly aid the nurse in addressing such ambiguity in reflection and discussion.

A two-day workshop has been developed at Reaside Clinic to assist in the development of clinical supervision skills, and all nursing staff are encouraged to attend. Nursing/care assistants are also encouraged to attend these workshops. This investment in care staff is designed to generate a culture of reflective practice in what has been recognised as a very demanding and challenging care environment.

Post-registration forensic nurse education

Formal, post-registration forensic nurse education has evolved over the past fifteen years in what can be viewed as a mirror to the service and clinical development in practice. The short course based on the principles of psychiatric nursing within secure environments (Joint Board of Clinical Nursing Studies [JBCNS] Course Number 960) was a course of four to six weeks' length. The aims of the course were to facilitate and enable an appreciation of the philosophy of care in secure environments, and to further enable nurses to plan and develop the nursing components of a multidisciplinary approach to managing therapeutic programmes within such settings. Nurses who completed this course were awarded a statement of attendance by the JBCNS. This course displayed a clear developmental path in terms of syllabuses and course breadth as compared to the earlier JBCNS course, which was based on care of the violent, or potentially violent, individual (Course Number 955). As with the JBCNS 960, the 955 course was also awarded with a certificate of attendance.

The English National Board (ENB) can be seen as responding to forensic service development and educational requirements again in 1988 in developing syllabuses for the nursing within controlled environments course (ENB 770). This course outlined what were distinct learning and teaching aims related to care of the mentally disordered offender in secure settings. The course outline made specific reference to developing and adapting present skill and acquiring new skills. Significantly reference was also made to extending the knowledge base within the field of practice. The course was openly innovative, at the time, in its length (six to nine months), and in its assessment criteria, which were continuous, both summative and formative, incorporating a clinical placement. Ashworth Special Hospital in Merseyside, and Reaside Medium Secure Unit in Birmingham, were the first hospitals to run this course in England. The creative ways in which facilitators approached this course proved to be encouraging to students examining their own attitudes in relation to their practice. Students certainly on the course at Birmingham in the early 1990s negotiated clinical placements in secure settings in Ireland, Canada and Holland, and others forged links with prison establishments and secure hospital environments around the United Kingdom. Formal visits to other secure hospital environments were made and students made formal and informal academic presentations as part of the course. There was an increased range of both summative and formative assessments within the course design. Thus the course was facilitating exposure and networking processes essential to the establishment and dissemination of newly acquired knowledge. Students' choice of clinical placements reflected closely what Mason and Mercer (1998) referred to as the heritage of forensic practice, policing, criminology and penology. Students were encouraged to complete small-scale research projects as part of the course requirement, and were supported in making their own choice of subjects to study. Interestingly, their choices reflected many of the areas which Kirby and Maguire later identified as constituting the work of the forensic psychiatric nurse: 'forensic environments', 'offending behaviour' and 'crime and the Forensic Psychiatric Nurse' and examples of nursing interventions (Kirby and Maguire, 1997, p. 395).

Higher education/links with the university sector

That post-registration nurse education was to move entirely into the university sector can be seen as being heralded by the changes to pre-registration nurse education, which occurred from 1986 onwards. Project 2000 (UKCC, 1986) effectively changed the status of nurses in 'training' to that of students in a higher education establishment. Pre-registration nurse education was now awarded at diploma and degree level. Post-registration courses offered at certificate level, whilst offering a Foundation level introduction to a subject, were viewed by some as less attractive than entering into studies at level 3 or above. Carton (1998) has gone further in specifically asking whether forensic certificate course provision met the 'challenge facing practitioners regarding advanced knowledge and skill development' (Carton, 1998, p. 252).

Such challenges, as stated earlier, related directly to service provision, the acquiring of new knowledge, and the wish to share such knowledge in a structured format delivered in an environment fostering discussion and debate. Modern universities adapted well to such developments, recognising that, with support, clinicians could develop areas of their work to enable others to acquire knowledge, attitudes and skill to function effectively in groundbreaking practice. This was the rationale behind the development of the sub-certificate course related to care of the mentally disordered offender in diversion services (ENB N56). Collaborative work between the English National Board, the University of Central England and Reaside Medium Secure Unit in Birmingham resulted in the delivery of a modular course which variously examined models of diverting the mentally disordered offender from the criminal justice system, related ethical and legal issues, as well as theoretical and practical applications. Here then was a course directly linked to secure provision in forensic practice. Elsewhere in the UK medium and maximum secure units were forging strong links with the university sector, notably Rampton Hospital and Sheffield Hallam University, Reaside Clinic and Birmingham University, the Hutton Centre and Teesside University and Ashworth Hospital and Liverpool University, to name but a few.

Such moves were clearly indicative of the need to encapsulate the rapid development and innovative service delivery in forensic practice, and marry this with appropriately framed education and training to advance and evaluate interventions and service delivery at the same time. Thus, in 1995 the medium secure providers in Birmingham in the form of Reaside Clinic developed a forensic psychiatric nursing pathway, which incorporated the ENB 770 course and the Higher Award, within a Post Experience Diploma and Masters in Science (P.Dip. MSc) course with the University of Birmingham. This course was specifically designed with nurses in mind, but was open to a range of professionals working in the field who could evidence their involvement in forensic practice to the university. This then enabled them to complete the two practice modules, integral to the forensic pathway of the course. The course had two parts; a Post Experience Diploma in Health Sciences (Specialist Practice), and the ENB Higher Award which comprised twelve modules in total, and a second part; Masters in Science (MSc) (Advanced Practice), and ENB Higher Award, which entailed completion of a further six modules to achieve the MSc. The course was offered on a full and part time basis.

Box 7.1 gives a list of the modules for the P.Dip. Health Sciences, which is clearly illustrative of the range of areas felt appropriate to a more comprehensive study of health science. The forensic individual clinical pathway constitutes a quarter of the first year of study. However students from forensic hospital settings were encouraged to make reference to their own practice in studying many of the year 1 modules. Within the course handbook specific reference is made to the work of Dewey (1916), who proposed education as a 'Process of reorganising experiences through which the individual is able to develop meaning and increase his/her control over the direction of his/her future experiences' (University of Birmingham, 1997).

This process of reconstruction of current social norms and practices is encouraged in higher education, to further encourage the student to examine their own belief and value systems. This is clearly outlined within the course literature. It was a clear indicator, as was the growth of similar courses in the study of mentally disordered offender groups, that educationalists were assisting the development of forensic psychiatric nursing as a speciality. The course was structured so as to contribute directly to practice development via protocol review, and contributed significantly to the forensic nursing knowledge base through the completion of a research dissertation in year 2. The pathways-specific modules, modules 4 and 5, addressed areas ranging from anger management, the psychology of behaviour and crime and mental disorder, to nursing diagnosis and evaluation of processes in practice. The assessment scheme was varied and utilised viva voce and unseen written examination, as well as submission of essays and a practice portfolio, as a requirement of the ENB Higher Award.

Educational course development in forensic practice in the early 1990s was beginning, but only beginning, to match service development. As

Grounds *et al.* (1993) noted, 'as a relatively new speciality, clinical growth in forensic psychiatry has tended to outstrip academic growth' (Grounds *et al.*, 1993, p. 729).

Many academic centres were leaning toward more broad based courses related to the study of the mentally disordered offender, as evidenced in developments at Birmingham University's Schools of Medicine, Psychology and Liverpool University. Such developments in course provision enabled a range of professionals allied to forensic psychiatric practice, nurses, police, social workers, psychologists and occupational therapists, to access the same course. This form of educational design and provision would appear to be the standard for future progression in this field. Forensic psychiatric practice and nursing has certainly had its critics and encountered much professional and public debate in recent decades. Much of this criticism has been deserved but it is gratifying to note that service managers and educationalists alike are addressing aspects of negative culture and practice, as Beacock (1994) identified:

That such issues are being addressed already is without doubt. The continued efforts of managers and educationalists in forensic settings has led to the development of meaningful multidisciplinary programmes of post basic education and an increasing awareness of the need to confront negative cultural norms. (Beacock, 1994, p. 542)

Box 7.1 Modules for the P.Dip Health Science (Specialist Practice)

ENB Higher Award Year 1
- Module 1 (c) Research Methods
- Module 2 (c) Statistics and Information Technology
- Module 3 (c) Health and Illness in Contemporary Society
- Module 4 (p) Bio/Psycho/Medical Sciences/Underpinning individual clinical pathway
- Module 5 (p) Assessment, Evaluation and Nursing Diagnostics
- Module 6 (c) Law and Ethics and Professional Practice
- Module 7 (c) Social Policy and the new NHS
- Module 8 (c) Human Systems and Change Processes
- Module 9 (p) Specialist Practice Clinical Fieldwork
- Module 10 (c) Evaluation, Quality and Audit
- Module 11 (p) Clinical Decision Making Skills/Clinical Fieldwork
- Module 12 (c) Practice Innovation Proposal

Key: c = core module; p = individual clinical pathway.
Source: The University of Birmingham, School of Health Science, Consultant Preceptor Handbook (1997)

The development of academic departments and the appointment of personnel related to education in forensic psychiatric practice can be seen as attributable to the vision of a small number of charismatic product champions. Such individuals are, and have been, extremely valuable in terms of encouraging academic institutions to recruit lecturers, lecturer/

practitioners and researchers with specific remits related to forensic psychiatric nursing, and behavioural science and practice. However, perhaps it is now time for the professionals involved in this area of practice to push for a forensic psychiatric standard, in relation to the curricula of both undergraduate and postgraduate mental health

References

Addo, Mary A. (2000) The role of the forensic nurse in clinical supervision. In David Robinson and Alyson Kettles (eds), *Forensic Nursing and Multidisciplinary Care of the Mentally Disordered Offender*. Jessica Kingsley, London, ch. 11.

Beacock, Colin (1994) A journey without end. Creating a development strategy for staff in secure forensic settings. In Tony Thompson and Peter Mathias (eds), *Lyttle's Mental Health and Disorder*, 2nd edn. Balliere Tindall, London, p. 542.

Carton, Gerry (1998) Nurse education: scribes and scriptures. In Tom Mason and Dave Mercer (eds), *Critical Perspectives in Forensic Care: Inside Out*. Macmillan, London, p. 252.

Collins, M. (2000) The practitioner new to the role of forensic psychiatric nurse in the UK. In David Robinson and Alyson Kettles (eds), *Forensic Nursing and Multidisciplinary Care of the Mentally Disordered Offender*. Jessica Kinglsey, London, ch. 3.

Dewey, J. (1916) *Democracy and Education*. The Free Press, New York (Cited in University of Birmingham (1997) School of Health Sciences (Nursing) Consultant Preceptor Handbook, PDip MSc Health Sciences.)

Grounds, Adrian, Snowden, Pete and Taylor, Pamela J. (1993) Forensic psychiatry in the National Health Service of England and Wales. In John Gunn and Pamela J. Taylor (eds), *Forensic Psychiatry – Clinical Legal and Ethical Issues* (1995 edition). Butterworth-Heinemann, Oxford, ch. 18.

Kettles, A.M. and Robinson, D.K. (2000) Overview and contemporary issues in the role of the forensic nurse in the UK. In David Robinson and Alyson Kettles (eds), *Forensic Nursing and Multidisciplinary Care of the Mentally Disordered Offender*. Jessica Kingsley, London, ch. 2.

Kettles, A.M. and Robinson, D.K. (1998) The lost vision of nursing. *Psychiatric Care*, 3 (4), pp. 126–9.

Kirby, S. and Maguire, N. (1997) Forensic psychiatric nursing. In Ben Thomas, Sally Hardy and Penny Cutting (eds), *Stuart and Sundeen's Mental Health Nursing Principles and Practice*. Mosby, London, ch. 26.

Mercer, Dave and Mason, Tom (1998) From devilry to diagnosis. The painful birth of forensic psychiatry. In Tom Mason and Dave Mercer (eds), *Critical Perspectives in Forensic Care: Inside Out*. Macmillan, London, ch. 2.

Proctor, B. (1988) Supervision: a co-operative exercise in accountability. In M. Marken and M. Payne (eds), *Enabling and Ensuring: Supervision in Practice*, 2nd edn. Leicester National Youth Bureau and Council for Education and Training in Youth and Community Work, pp. 21–34.

Storey, L. and Dale, C. (1999) Nursing in Secure Environments Scoping Study. United Kingdom Central Council for Nursing, Midwifery and Health Visiting and the University of Central Lancashire. UKCC, London.

United Kingdom Central Council for Nursing, Midwifery and Health Visiting (UKCC) (1986) *Project 2000: A New Preparation for Practice*. UKCC, London.

United Kingdom Central Council for Nursing Midwifery and Health Visiting (UKCC) (1995) *Initial Position Statement on Clinical Supervision*. UKCC, London.

University of Birmingham School of Health Sciences (Nursing) Consultant Preceptor Handbook. PE Dip/MSc Health Sciences.

Diversion from custody

Stuart Wix and Hayley Cushing

Introduction

Diversion of mentally disordered offenders (MDOs) from the criminal justice system has become an accepted principle of care over the past ten years within the United Kingdom (Blumenthal and Wessley, 1992). There has been a large investment in diversion services for MDOs and forensic psychiatry during this time. Programmes have sought to address the plight of the mentally ill at all stages of the criminal justice system, at police stations, magistrates courts and prison, by placing individuals more appropriately into the care of health and social services. The establishment of diversion services can also be set against fundamental changes of approach by mental health services in recent years, which have become more community focused, and an increase in public concern, where high profile cases with tragic consequences have led to a series of inquiries (see Ritchie Report, 1994).

In 1995 the Home Office estimated that there were approximately 100 multi-agency diversion assessment schemes in operation, which predominantly involved forensic psychiatric services. Provision of comprehensive diversion services offers benefits for the mentally disordered who come into conflict with the law, as well as those otherwise involved in the process, including the police, Crown Prosecution Service and courts. The aim is to give access to the most appropriate disposal for this potentially vulnerable group.

Diversion at the point of arrest: diversion from the police station

In contrast to how offenders usually enter the criminal justice system, following arrest and charging at a police station, court assessment schemes had commonly preceded the establishment of diversion at the point of arrest services and shown encouraging results in reducing the need for remand in custody for the mentally disordered offender (James and Hamilton, 1992; Holloway and Shaw, 1992; Exworthy and Parrott, 1993; Pierzchniak *et al.*, 1997). It was, however, widely recognised that a significant number of individuals who had been screened at court, may have spent a considerable time in custody (Laing, 1995). The natural progression and extension of the court diversion scheme was to make psychiatric assessment available at police stations (Wix, 1994).

Piloting the service

The first recognised scheme in the United Kingdom was a one-year pilot project introduced at Bournville Lane police station in Birmingham. The pilot project was regarded as highly successful and was extended to include four more police stations in the south of the city. Other forensic mental health services viewed the service as a 'blueprint' and adopted similar police station assessment schemes around the country, with particular emphasis being placed upon busy city areas.

The main aim of diversion at the point of arrest (DAPA) is to ensure that mentally disordered offenders receive prompt care and treatment in the appropriate setting, avoiding potentially harmful periods in custody. They offer police stations the services of a community psychiatric nurse (CPN) 24 hours per day, seven days a week. If called to assess someone the CPN obtains all the relevant information from the arresting officer before interviewing the individual concerned. Screening is designed to determine whether or not there are particular mental health problems and assess the presence of serious mental illness and associated risks of potential self-harm, harm to others or suicide. The CPN acts as the co-ordinator for the involvement of other mental health workers and services where required.

After assessment, the CPN will discuss an offender's mental state with the custody officer, the police surgeon, arresting officer if available, and the duty inspector for those who are identified as mentally ill. They might then recommend hospital admission and treatment, or arrange psychiatric outpatient appointments. Individuals might also be referred to community based services such as a day centre.

If the offender is assessed as suffering from a mental health problem and only faces charges for a minor offence, and where some appropriate alternative to prosecution are available, it is often perceived not to be in the public interest to pursue prosecution.

Police and Criminal Evidence Act (PACE) 1984

Mental health professionals who provide services to police stations will benefit from a working knowledge of PACE, given the impact it has upon individuals detained in police custody.

An individual who is detained at a police station having been arrested has the following rights:

- to be told why they are detained;
- to have someone informed about their whereabouts;
- to obtain free legal advice, and in particular to have a solicitor present during questioning;
- to request a medical examiner;
- for information passed to the 'appropriate adult' to be treated in confidence;
- to have an interpreter if they cannot understand English.

The role of the forensic medical examiner (FME)

2. The custody officer must immediately call the police surgeon if a person brought to a police station or already detained there:
(a) appears to be suffering from a mental disorder/handicap...(Police and Criminal Evidence Act 1984)

The role of the forensic medical examiner (FME) in relation to mentally disordered offenders is clearly defined by PACE. When an individual is arrested for an offence and where mental disorder is suspected an FME will assess to establish whether or not the person is:

(a) Fit to be detained?
(b) Fit to be interviewed/questioned?

Prior to the establishment of CPN assessment schemes at police stations, custody officers were entirely reliant upon the services and assessment skills of FMEs. A number of difficulties existed with this arrangement, including a big spending shortage on FMEs approved under Section 12 (2) of the Mental Health Act 1983. The quality of the mental state examination was also brought into question. This concern was highlighted by Gudjunssen (1992), who carried out a survey within the Metropolitan Police Authority, and found that only 9.5 per cent of FMEs were approved under Section 12 (2). FMEs are not a distinct professional group, often being general practitioners. In some instances FMEs have welcomed the presence of a CPN, and estimated a significant fall in mental health referrals by as much as 95 per cent (Wix, 1994).

The key strategy for using forensic CPNs in establishing early assessment services was based upon knowledge of the criminal justice system, an established network of health and social service contacts across districts, and an ability to facilitate non-custodial and social care options where available. In recent years, increasing numbers of DAPA services have been led by generic CPN teams or jointly managed by acute and forensic services.

The aims of police station assessment services are to:

- Provide better and more comprehensive assessments at police stations.
- Provide improved access to mental health and alternative services.
- Provide a more consistent service by key professionals.
- Provide follow-up care and support.
- Ensure better liaison between agencies.

Within the West Midlands the police themselves have also been interested and concerned about the numbers of mentally disordered offenders brought into police custody and in particular to investigate the operation of Section 136 of the Mental Health Act 1983. This allows the police the power to remove people believed to be suffering from a mental illness to a 'place of safety' for the purpose of psychiatric assessment.

Data were collected in a study of six police stations in the City of Birmingham in 1990. Roughton (1994) studied a total of 207 separate custody records relating to people detained under Section 136. The results showed that the majority of detainees were male and that the average time spent in custody was about 3 hours and 45 minutes. Forty-six per cent of the sample had previously been admitted to hospital either voluntarily or compulsorily, and 26 per cent were released from custody apparently unsupervised and unsupported.

Diversion at the point of arrest offers intervention at the earliest possible opportunity, providing rapid access to care and treatment if necessary. Identification of the mentally ill at this stage provides an opportunity for intervention at some later point, either at the time of their appearance at court or whilst on bail or remand in prison The Forensic CPN has been a key professional in pioneering the role of liaison, and the link person to accessing appropriate services. The presence of a DAPA service alongside court assessment schemes can enhance integrated diversion services.

Collaboration at the various stages of diversion ensures that MDOs are not lost within the criminal justice system and that appropriate care, support and treatment is maintained throughout.

Diversion from the magistrates court

Psychiatric services for mentally disordered offenders at the court stage have been in existence since 1985, when panel schemes were first established, in response to concern regarding the quality of psychiatric reports and offenders receiving inappropriate prison sentences (Staite *et al.*, 1994).

The North West Hertfordshire scheme, an experimental project, was led by a probation officer, and involved the co-ordination of a multi-agency panel meeting whenever a psychiatric report was requested by the court. The offender would be seen by health professionals such as a psychiatrist, psychologist, community psychiatric nurse and a social worker, who, with a probation officer, could plan a management strategy and package of care which would enable the individual to remain in the community. Although the quality of psychiatric reports and subsequent recommendations improved, panel schemes relied upon the goodwill of the professionals concerned, and lacked proper funding. As a result, very few such schemes are still in existence.

In 1990, the Home Office issued circular 66/90 which advocated that mentally disordered offenders in need of psychiatric care and treatment should receive assistance from health and social services wherever appropriate, and as soon as possible. The circular also stated that 'where this is not possible there should be provision for appropriate mental health care within police custody, transition through the courts and custody in prison whether remanded or convicted'.

In essence, this pointed to the urgent need for diversion services to be established within the criminal justice system and recommended a complete review in order to implement radical changes. Since that time there have been more than 100 diversion schemes developed in England and Wales.

There was mounting concern regarding the increasing prison population and the numbers of inmates committing suicide or involved in acts of self-harm within prisons (Woolf Report and Tumin Report, Home Office, 1990).

The Health of the Nation (Department of Health, 1992), which outlined targets to reduce the number of suicides in custody, reflected the concerns expressed by both Tumin and Woolf.

Court diversion schemes in England and Wales operate differently according to demographic factors, service provision, resourcing, and such factors as the number of police stations and courts within a particular area. The service requirements for a heavily populated city with a large network of police stations feeding into a busy central court will differ from a more rural area with fewer, smaller police stations and courts sitting only for a few sessions each week. Schemes in various locations have been tailored to the requirements of each area. Some have developed on-call services, with a psychiatric nurse or psychiatrist serving one or more police stations and the related courts. Some of the busier city area schemes provide daily input to the main courts and have a pro-active approach.

The Birmingham service

An example of a pro-active service is the scheme which exists in the Victoria Law Courts, Birmingham. This houses the largest magistrates court system in Europe (Hillis, 1993). It has 24 courts with a varying number sitting at any one time. One of these is allocated to deal with arrests during the preceding twenty-four hours. A CFPN visits the cells every morning to scrutinise Crown Prosecution Service (CPS) files and screen out defendants who might require assessment. The general criteria for assessment include:

- Serious violence.
- Known/suspected psychiatric history.
- Drugs and/or alcohol use/dependence.
- Self-harm or suicidal behaviour.
- Odd or bizarre behaviour observed.
- Concern by police or others.

Once screening has taken place, an assessment is preceded by an explanation to the defendant, who is given the option to terminate the process should they not wish to proceed. Assessments generally take place in an interview room except when the defendant is disturbed, in which case the CFPN may conduct the interview in the cell.

Assessment is by way of a semi-structured interview and revolves around information gleaned from the CPS files. For the purpose of record keeping, some questions are factual, based particularly in relation to the defendant's own account of why they are subject to criminal proceedings, which will often lead the interview into other areas of concern. This process often provides indicators on which the CFPN can focus to gain a clearer picture of the mental state of the defendant. The assessment determines whether or not there is an identified mental disorder. Important areas of concern are the presence of disorders such as psychosis, depression and associated risks of potential self-harm and suicide. The nature of the assessment and screening process requires that the CFPN is responsible for making decisions in conjunction with the court probation officer regarding the formulation of appropriate recommendations to the court.

Role of the Crown Prosecutor

Assessments have to be completed within a limited timeframe in order to have any available recommendations formulated before court proceedings commence. In addition, discussion can take place with solicitors, medical staff and other services in order to check facts and obtain more detailed information. Important discussion can also take place between the probation officer, the CFPN and Crown Prosecutor before any recommendation is made to the court. The agreement of the Crown Prosecutor is vital from a legal standpoint, if successful diversion is to be achieved.

If the offence is of a serious nature, careful consideration must be given to the possible need for secure provision such as a psychiatric intensive care unit or admission to a medium secure unit. Discontinuance of proceedings cannot be considered at this stage, and may be postponed until a later point when the CPS have had more time to make an informed decision.

The CPS Annual Report 1995–1996 listed common public interest factors in favour of prosecution:

(a) The use of a weapon or violence during the commission of an offence.
(b) The offence was committed against a person serving the public (for example, a police or prison officer, or a nurse).
(c) The victim of the offence was vulnerable, has been put under considerable fear or suffered personal attack, damage or disturbance.
(d) The grounds of the offence are likely to be considered or repeated.

There are two factors that a crown prosecutor must take into account before a decision is made to prosecute:

1. At first there must be enough evidence for the case to progress, including witness and victim statements.
2. CPS will only start or continue to prosecute if it is in the public interest or there is enough evidence to provide realistic prospects of conviction.

If a prosecutor is given an assessment which indicates that a detainee is mentally disordered and in need of psychiatric treatment, he/she may be more likely to consider diversion with or without conditions of bail if the charge or nature of the offence warrants this course of action.

Court probation officer

The majority of well established diversion services at magistrates courts rely upon close liaison between health care professionals and the court based probation team. There may be an identified probation officer with a specific remit for mental health liaison. The probation officer can therefore assist the CPN with regard to advice on court procedure and protocol. The probation officer can also assist in the follow-up of defendants where a psychiatric report is requested and make the necessary arrangements with a local psychiatrist and community mental health teams to ensure that this task is completed.

Probation officers are also key in co-ordinating regular meetings between court personnel (CPS, solicitors, security staff etc.) and mental health workers involved in providing a diversion service. Regular meetings between participating agencies, offer a platform to 'iron out' problems and agree service objectives and policy. Staite *et al.* (1994) recommend that members of such groups should be senior enough to operate efficiently at a strategic multi-agency level, and possess a good understanding of the criminal justice system as a whole.

In addition to the probation officer, a bail information officer can assist the process of diversion by co-ordinating a set of arrangements which make the granting of bail more likely.

The probation service has an important role to play in assisting the process of identifying individuals who may need attention at a later date, and aiding the diversion of defendants from custody to appropriate health care provision alongside CPN colleagues.

Diversion from prison

Empirical studies during the past ten years have shown that the prevalence of mental disorder in the prison population is high (Gunn, 1987; Grounds, 1990).

The Reed Report (Department of Health and the Home Office, 1992) highlighted the need for an efficient process of diverting mentally disordered offenders in custody to appropriate services, particularly for those on remand. Prison diversion schemes, which are also regarded as the 'third safety net', have evolved out of the perceived need to bridge the gap between individuals being diverted and finally linked in to appropriate health care services. A survey undertaken in Birmingham in 1992 showed that of 60 Special Hospital referrals, as many as two-thirds had been involved with the criminal justice system prior to the index offence. This would suggest that for some offending behaviour may escalate mental health problems that are not detected. Transfers from prison to hospital for prisoners on remand can be made under Section 47 or 48 of the Mental Health Act 1983.

A solution to the problem

Funding for health workers with a remit to screen and assess newly remanded defendants has come from a variety of combined sources. Psychiatric nurses have often been identified as the natural choice to fulfil this role. This has been reflected in prison diversion schemes around the country. In the Birmingham scheme, which has been based at Winson Green Prison since 1993, a project worker was employed to provide short term support for prisoners diverted from custody until an appropriate package of care could be negotiated with outside services. The project worker would also carry out mental health screening of newly remanded prisoners as they were processed on. The role of this individual has evolved over time through a process of networking around the institution and by making the service an integral part of the system.

Reception area

The first point of contact with individuals when they arrive at the prison is the reception officer, whose task is to confirm factual details and to confirm the decision of the court. A record is made of personal effects and any other relevant information. A health care officer observes and assesses the prisoner, highlighting any areas of physical or psychological need.

Mental health screening

The diversion support worker (DSW) screens prisoners based on information already gleaned from the mental health screening interview at the court stage. Following discussions with bail information services, a decision may be made on the best course to follow. Local services and the individual's GP may be contacted immediately in order to obtain details regarding previous contact, treatment and so on in order to assist in providing the most appropriate form of care. Occasionally, a prisoner may be identified as at risk of potential suicide or self-harm. Interviews are conducted in an informal manner, given the constraints and surroundings of the prison environment. When a mental health problem is suspected later referrals for assessment can be taken from prison officers and other agencies within the prison.

The DSW may liaise with and offer advice to probation services, as well as hostel staff within the prison catchment area. The presence of a DSW offers the opportunity to facilitate and increase awareness of mental health issues among prison officers and other professionals within the prison.

Evaluation of the service

The overall aims of the service are:

1. To identify mental health problems among remand prisoners at the earliest possible opportunity.
2. To pro-actively facilitate diversion within and from custody.

During the first two years of the Birmingham scheme during which a psychiatric nurse was available to the prison, approximately 1700 newly remanded prisoners were assessed as suffering from some form of mental disorder. Twenty-five per cent of this group required immediate transfer to the prison health care centre. The remainder required interventions that included multi-cell occupation, for instance where suicidal ideas had been expressed. Other prisoners were referred to drug and alcohol agencies and groups, or for stress management. The input from the DSW was seen as benefiting patients, the prison service and the community, and has become an essential component of an integrated network of diversion services.

Diversion in action: Elliott House

Courts in the past have been faced with the dilemma of what to do with defendants who have been charged with offences which might lead to a community disposal or custodial sentence who may also be suffering from a mental disorder. Elliott House was until recently the only specialised statutory bail and probation hostel in the country for residents with this sort of problem. It was established in Birmingham, in 1993, as a partnership between the West Midlands Probation Service (WMPS) and the Regional Forensic Psychiatric Service based at Reaside Clinic. Elliott House is a national resource attracting referrals from all over England and Wales of those who require mental health support. Prior to it opening in 1993, a multiprofessional group developed the good notion of partnership between probation and a health services. Good working relationships led to the development of Elliott House.

The need for specialist accommodation for the mentally disordered offender whilst awaiting trial or sentencing had already been highlighted, as a high proportion of mentally disordered offenders were homeless. The emergence of an approved specialised hostel appeared to be appropriate. The collaborative inter-agency working between the probation service and the regional forensic services fulfilled a key principle of the 1997 Department of Health White Paper which considered that the NHS should work in partnership with other agencies to put the needs of patients at the centre of the care process.

Elliott House was originally a voluntary approved probation hostel run by a management committee. More recently the probation service took ownership. It is a male-only hostel with space for twenty residents. It is centrally funded. The staff group consists of two qualified senior probation officers, one of whom is the hostel manager and the other is deputy manager. The remaining staff are unqualified. There are six day assistant wardens and two night assistant wardens. There is an office administrator and a housekeeper who manages domestic staff who provide full catering and cleaning facilities, although the residents are encouraged to do their own washing and ironing.

As with other approved hostels there is no requirement for the probation staff to have any specific mental health training or prior experience. Some training has, nevertheless, been provided with informal sessions, which have been staff-led. Generally information provided by the referring CPN or probation officer should indicate that the prospective resident is suffering from a treatable mental disorder and that evidence exists of a psychiatric history and or previous contact with local services.

Those with primary drug/alcohol problems, or those suffering from a personality disorder, cannot be accepted, along with those whose mental illness is acute enough to warrant admission to hospital. Individuals whose sole diagnosis is of a learning difficulty are less likely to be accepted, although consideration would be given to a person who was also believed to be suffering with a treatable mental illness. Acceptance of this type of referral would also be more likely where the severity of the learning disability was felt to be manageable in the setting of a probation hostel.

Referral process

Referrals are taken over the telephone by an assistant warden. As much information as possible is sought, including demographic data, offence-related details and the most up to date psychiatric information. This can take the form of a CPN assessment, or psychiatric or psychology reports. Information from a non-health professional alone may be insufficient. Once a decision to accept the individual is made, the issue of a suitable curfew for a potential resident is raised. This may be in excess of that set by a mainstream bail hostel, due to consideration of the degree of illness and nature of the alleged offence. Tighter curfews are helpful in observation of a resident's mental state in the early phase. Key workers and residents will have weekly supervision sessions together, with all information gathered being examined in deciding what recommendation should be contained within the pre-schedule report. Psychiatric reports may also have been requested by the courts. These can be undertaken at Elliott House. Recommendations or findings are discussed in full at the weekly multi-disciplinary meeting held at the hostel. A plan of action can then be formulated and a future package of appropriate care and treatment agreed.

On arrival at Elliott House the resident is taken through an induction process by the assistant warden on duty. Information given includes hostel rules, daily timetables and some idea of the residents' general expectations. Information gathered by staff include next of kin, benefits claimed or employment details and information on current medication, mental and physical health and any risk of self-harm or suicide. If there is any immediate cause for concern the CFPN is contacted and a full evaluation made.

The role of the CFPN is to see new residents and complete a full mental health assessment. The CFPN would then refer the individual to medical colleagues or identify those residents who do not require psychiatric intervention. The level of suicide/self-harm risk is also assessed for each individual.

Local services are routinely contacted to confirm previous psychiatric history and plans of care, and, if appropriate, to maintain links whilst the resident remains on bail at the hostel. Assistant warden staff at the hostel are also appraised of recommended general management strategies and advised of how new residents' immediate needs might best be met. Following the CFPN assessment a member of the medical team will assess the resident and prescribe medication if required and formulate an initial treatment plan. Assistant wardens perform the role of keyworker to each resident. A full risk assessment is undertaken, according to a model devised by the West Midlands Probation Service. Each resident is subject to regular multi-disciplinary and inter-agency review.

Both medical and nursing staff provide a 24-hour on-call service to the hostel where advice can be given or further assessment sought. The occupational therapist provides social skills training, drug awareness training and a variety of other forms of input. A clinical psychologist provides input where appropriate. The initial length of stay at Elliott House is dependent on the needs of the resident. When it is felt that the resident should move on, full support is provided for the individual to settle into any new environment and to ensure that full psychiatric and social support are in place. Some residents do return to Elliott House if they are placed on a probation order with a condition of residence and/or treatment.

Facts and figures

Geelan *et al.* (1998), in describing the work of Elliott House, highlighted a number of interesting findings. Data were collected between August 1994 and April 1996 and a total of 83 cases were analysed. Forty-seven per cent of the residents had a psychotic disorder. Seventy-four per cent had had previous contact with psychiatric services, and 54 per cent were of no fixed abode. Ninety-nine per cent were unemployed. Even with the high rate of psychiatric morbidity, unemployment and homelessness, only 6 per cent were in contact with social services. The authors suggest that there is 'an association between a breakdown in contact with psychiatric and social services and offending in such individuals' (Geelan *et al.*, 1998, p. 105).

Thirty per cent of residents originated from outside the West Midlands region, and 41 per cent from outside the West Midlands Probation Service area. There may be considerable benefit in future in providing more localised services.

Conclusion

Elliott House demonstrates that it is possible to provide a specialised approved hostel for the mentally disordered offender. It also shows that a close partnership between separately managed agencies can successfully provide a high level of care for this vulnerable group of people. Elliott House has clearly prevented a significant number of mentally disordered offenders from being remanded into custody and has provided a positive alternative to custody by offering realistic community based disposals for the courts.

It has been acknowledged that Elliott House is a pro-active approach to the plight of mentally disordered offenders in certain circumstances, and based upon its success has led to proposals to fund a further two hostels in the London and Manchester areas respectively, based on the Elliott House model.

Why divert?

The question of whether to divert and why forensic services have been pivotal in the provision of such services has been debated throughout the 1990s. Chung *et al.* (1998) has argued that diversion schemes led by forensic services may not be the most economic set-up. Thomas-Peter and Oliver (2000) have also highlighted a dramatic rise in capital expenditure, and indicated that forensic services have failed to demonstrate an equal level of increase in effectiveness in diverting the mentally abnormal offenders from the criminal justice system. Increased provision for diversion from custody leads to an increase in expenditure and need for increased funding. This often brings apparently improved provision and leads to a decline in numbers of mentally abnormal offenders seen in some areas of the criminal justice system and the perception that the service is over-staffed or too lavishly funded. To concentrate solely on the funding and cost of such services would be to miss the point of diversion, and risks ignoring the literature which has highlighted the increasing numbers of mentally ill who have become unnecessarily incarcerated in penal establishments. It can therefore be argued that the concept of diversion offers a compassionate method of dealing with mentally disordered offenders.

Prins (1992) takes a different perspective when considering the efficacy of diversion. He asks the question whether some mentally disordered offenders would prefer to be prosecuted in the normal way, as opposed to being labelled with a psychiatric diagnosis? He also raises the dilemma of whether to pursue prosecution or divert from custody and whether a mentally disordered individual can or should be held responsible for their actions. He also argues that because a diversion service is focused upon the welfare of a mentally disordered offender, little or no consideration may be given to the victim.

Although these are only some of the concerns raised in relation to diversion from custody, it is important for those involved in diversion services to be aware of them. They offer a means of enhancing practice and remaining focused upon the job in hand. Critical analysis of the role of the Community Psychiatric Nurse in diversion remains an important component in development of services. The need for continuing evaluation and research remains.

Conclusion and evaluation

The principle of diverting mentally abnormal offenders from custody to secure the most appropriate care and treatment or help from social services, is in essence a sound one. There is a diversity of provision, at present reflecting variation in who takes lead role as well as in the method of operation. Different schemes for diversion have developed in keeping with local need and variation. The most commonly adopted models are pro-active, often led by CPNs and located in city and suburban areas. Such services often develop into an integrated network of options involving assessment at police stations, in courts and prisons and in probation hostels.

Diversion schemes aim to find a solution to the problem of mentally disordered offenders caught up in the criminal justice system. Research has clearly demonstrated the effectiveness of this approach in terms of identifying offenders with mental health problems (James, 1996; Riordan and Wix, 2000), reducing the period of custody between arrest and hospital based treatment (James and Hamilton, 1992) and providing a realistic community based alternative (Exworthy and Parrott, 1993).

It is important to acknowledge that diversion from custody to health care provision is not always successful. A defendant's progress may be hindered due to the court's rejection of a bail application or where mental health services are unable to provide a suitable immediate response. This does not necessarily indicate failure but may be due to circumstances beyond the control of those agencies involved in attempting to divert a defendant. Diversion services can only be successful when a multi-agency approach is adopted with a shared vision and purpose.

References

Blumenthal, S. and Wessley, S. (1992) National survey of current arrangements for diversion from custody in England and Wales. *British Medical Journal*, 305, pp. 1322–5.

Chung, M.C., Cumella, S., Wensley, J. and Easthope, Y. (1998) A description of a forensic service in one city in the United Kingdom. *Medicine Science and the Law*. 38, pp. 242–50.

Chung, M.C., Cumella, S., Wensley, J. and Easthope, Y. (1999) A follow-up study of mentally disordered offenders after a court diversion scheme: six-month and one year comparison. *Medicine Science and the Law*, 38, 31–7.

Department of Health (1992) *The Health of the Nation: A Strategy for Health in England*. London: HMSO.

Department of Health and the Home Office (1992) *Review of Health and Social Services for Mentally Disordered Offenders and Others Requiring Similar Services* (The Reed Report). HMSO, London.

Department of Health (1997) *The New NHS: Modern, Dependable*. (CM 3897), HMSO, London.

Exworthy, T. and Parrott, J. (1993) Evaluation of a diversion from custody scheme at magistrates courts. *Journal of Forensic Psychiatry*, 4, pp. 497–505.

Farrar, M. (1996) Government policy on mentally disordered offenders and its implementation. *Journal of Mental Health*, 2, pp. 224–33.

Geelan, S., Griffin, N. and Briscoe, J. (1998) A profile of residents at Elliott House, the first approved bail hostel and probation hostel specifically for mentally disordered offenders. *Health Trends*, 30, pp. 102–5.

Grounds, A. (1990) Transfers of sentenced prisoners to hospitals. *Criminal Law Review*, pp. 545–51.

Gudjunssen, G. (1992) *The Psychology of Interrogation: Confessions and Testimony*. Chichester: Wiley.

Hillis, G. (1993) Diverting tactics. *Nursing Times*, 89 (1), pp. 24–7.

Holloway, J. and Shaw, J. (1992) Providing a forensic service to a magistrates court. *Journal of Forensic Psychiatry*, 3, pp. 153–9.

Home Office (1990) Prison Disturbances, April 1990: Report of an Inquiry by Rt Hon. Lord Justice Woolf (Parts I and II) and His Honour Judge Stephen Tumin (Part II). Cmnd 1456, London HMSO.

James, A. (1996) *Life on the Edge. Diversion and the Mentally Disordered Offender*. Mental Health Foundation, London.

James, D.V. and Hamilton, L.N. (1992) Setting up psychiatric liaison schemes to magistrates courts, probation and practicalities. *Medicine Science and the Law*, 32, pp. 167–76.

Joseph, P. and Potter, M. (1993) Diversion from custody, 1. Psychiatric assessment at the magistrates court. *British Journal of Psychiatry*, 162, pp. 325–30.

Laing, J.M. (1995) The mentally disordered suspect at the police station. *Criminal Law Review*, pp. 371–9.

Pierzchniak, P., Purchase, N. and Kennedy, H. (1997) Liaison between prison, court and psychiatric services. *Health Trends*, 29, pp. 26–9.

Prins, H. (1992) Diversion of the mentally disordered: some problems for criminal justice, penology and healthcare. *Journal of Forensic Psychiatry*, 3(3), pp. 431–43.

Riordan, S. and Wix, S. (1999) Diversion of mentally disordered offenders to what and when? *British Journal of Forensic Practice*, 2, pp. 23–6.

Ritchie Report (1994) Factors Influencing the Implementation of the Care Programme Approach. Research Study carried out for the Department of Health by Social and

Community Planning Research. London, HMSO.

Roughton, A. (1994) An Investigation into the Operation of Section 136 of the Mental Health Act 1983 in the West Midlands. Report to the West Midlands Police.

Staite, C., Martin, N. Bingham, M. and Daly, R. (1994) Diversion from Custody for Mentally Disordered Offenders. Langman, London.

Thomas-Peter, B. and Oliver, C. (2000) Diversion from Custody. Submitted for publication *Psychology and Politics Expert Evidence*.

Wix, S. (1994) Keeping on the straight and narrow. Diversion at the point of arrest. *Psychiatric Care*, July/August, pp. 102–4.

Aftercare

Richard Carter, Gina Hillis and Andy Hunt

Some professionals feel that the appropriate focus of care within a medium secure setting reflects the ability, or not, of the patient to function effectively within a community setting. Many philosophies of care within medium secure establishments incorporate concepts associated with 'normalisation'. This 'normalisation' can be interpreted as how ready a patient is for discharge, and how well they may fit into a community setting. The decisions and processes associated with this particular area comprise one of the most crucial aspects of patient care, and this chapter intends to provide a brief overview of some of the reports and inquiries involving the care of mentally disordered offenders which often have a direct impact upon decisions made to move patients towards discharge and community care. The chapter will also reflect the process of moving the patient on to the community, and will utilise two case studies to further illustrate this.

Reports and inquiries into the care of mentally disordered offenders

Whilst many of the reports and inquiries of the past decade may imply some sort of causal link between crime and mental disorder, their remit is to explore the circumstances which surround particular events and to make recommendations for service improvements and policy regarding mentally disordered offenders. Policy regarding care in the community has undergone many changes in the light of such inquiries and affects both restriction order patients as well as non-restriction order patients. In examining many more of the recent inquiries, particularly the Ritchie Report (Ritchie *et al.*, 1994) and 'The Falling Shadow' (Blom-Cooper *et al.*, 1995), there has been much more debate about programmes associated with care in the community, particularly in relation to mentally disordered offenders.

The Ritchie Report investigated the care and treatment of Christopher Clunis, who had a diagnosis of paranoid schizophrenia. He made an unprovoked attack which caused the death of Jonathan Zito in a London underground station. This particular case sharply brought into focus the psychiatric care of the severely mentally ill who are living in the community. The report commented extensively on supervision in the community and made twenty-six recommendations that have a direct impact on nursing care and the role of the multidisciplinary team in relation to community aftercare as well as the involvement of the police and the Crown Prosecution Service. The report questioned policies in place at the time, and amongst the most significant recommendations was the setting up of supervision registers of patients thought to be at particular risk of violence to others, or suicide or self-neglect.

The decision-making process regarding inclusion on the supervision register was incorporated into the process of the Care Programme Approach (Department of Health, 1990), as legislated within the National Health Service and Community Care Act 1990.

The notion of comprehensive risk assessments being incorporated into Care Programme Approach documentation was further echoed by Blom-Cooper *et al.* (1995) in 'The Falling Shadow'. This was a report of an inquiry into incidents involving a psychiatric patient called Andrew Robinson who stabbed an occupational therapist, Georgina Robinson (no relation), in Torquay, Devon. Crichton (1995a) examined the issues of risk of violence and its management in relation to this incident. Crichton (1995a) suggests that the longer term responses to risk are monitoring and supervision, which depends centrally on the maintenance of a relationship with the patient. Community psychiatric nurses are able to develop close working relationships with patients as they often have the most frequent contact with them, and Repper and Perkins (1995) suggest that CPNs concentrate on the development of long term, trusting and valuing relationships based upon positive, empathic understanding.

There have been several reports about violence committed by psychiatric patients following discharge from hospital. Amongst those publicised cases have been that of Sharon Campbell (Spokes *et al.*, 1988), Kevin Rooney (Collins *et al.*, 1994) and Michael Buchanan (Heginbotham *et al.*, 1994). None of these patients was under any statutory form of supervision or restriction whilst in the community. The report of the Independent Panel of Inquiry into the case of Jason Mitchell (Blom-Cooper *et al.*, 1996) made very detailed recommendations to be applied as a consequence of the case. Jason Mitchell was also under a restriction order on discharge, when he murdered his father and an elderly couple. This raises the question as to how effective the monitoring and supervision of those on a restriction order is in preventing further offending.

In the light of such reports there has been widespread concern about care in the community, particularly for mentally disordered offenders. Boyd estimated that twenty homicides a year are committed by psychiatric patients in England and Wales (Department of Health, 1996), but there is no way of knowing precisely how many acts of violence are committed by this group. The arrangements for cooperation between statutory agencies in the management of mentally disordered offenders are set out in Home Office Circular No. 66/90 (1990), which suggests that this patient group receive care and treatment from health and social services and not within the criminal justice system. The Reed Report (Department of Health and the Home Office, 1992) endorsed this view and enunciated five main guiding principles regarding quality of care for mentally disordered offenders. These principles were that care should be based on individual need and as far as possible be in the community near the patient's home. The level of security should be justified by the patient's dangerousness and, finally, care should be aimed at maximising rehabilitation and the prospect of independent living.

The Home Office Circular 66/90 and the Reed Report both contributed to Home Office circular 29/93, Community Care Reforms and the Criminal Justice System (Home Office, 1993), which drew attention to the role of the probation service and its involvement in provision in the community, particularly following release from prison, and also whilst on a probation order with a condition of treatment. Many mentally disordered offenders require treatment in hospital whilst serving a prison sentence and hence require admission to a medium secure unit. Some complete their sentence under a hospital order under the Mental Health Act 1983 and some will have an additional restriction order placed upon them. Some will return to prison to complete their sentence. The Hospital Direction, which has become known as the 'Hybrid Order', was suggested by the Working Group on Psychopathic Disorder (Home Office and Department of Health 1994. Here the proposal is that patients must return to prison when their mental illness was sufficiently treated, however, the report also indicated that a prisoner must return to hospital if their behaviour indicated psychological disturbance. In the case of psychopathic disorder this has resource implications, which will increase the demand on beds that are already under pressure to meet existing commitments. The treatability of this client group makes them a management concern within hospitals, as discussed by Blackburn (1992) and, also when planning discharge into the community.

In the case of patients with a psychiatric illness, a return to prison can mean disruption in treatment, the opportunity to avoid medication and hence, a deterioration in mental state. The situation is such that for patients going back to prison, as well as those coming back into hospital, care plans and continuity are both disrupted, significantly affecting assessments, particularly risk assessment, as discussed by Crichton (1995a).

This disruption in continuity of care can impair therapeutic relationships which are essential to maintain mentally disordered offenders when they return to the community, particularly when compliance with treatment is required. Coid (1991) highlights the question of whether people with serious mental illness should be in the community at all and criticises the relevance of community out-reach services for the subgroup of what has become known as the severely mentally ill.

The decision not to introduce community supervision orders by the House of Commons Health Committee (Home Office, 1993) expressed concern where mentally disordered offenders are non-compliant with treatment and the Supervised Discharge Act (Home Office, 1995) reflected that action be taken should this happen.

Supervised discharge came into force in April 1996, arising from the Mental Health (Patients in the Community) Act (Home Office, 1995). The named key worker is allowed a power to convey the patient, in order that examination for compulsory admission is carried out, including revisiting existing risk assessments. This differs from a restriction order, where the Home Office impose conditions upon the patient and will return the patient to hospital if he/she is non-compliant, if he /she offends or there is evidence of significant risk to the public.

A conditional discharge is the tightest community power over a patient according to Crichton (1995b). The patient can apply for absolute discharge from the restriction order but this is subject to the favourable reports from the social supervisor to the Home Office with evidence of compliance, and risk assessments, which must confirm that the patient no longer poses a threat to the public.

Community staff in medium secure units are involved in the provision of care of mentally disordered offenders as they progress towards discharge from hospital and to community placements. As members of a multi-disciplinary team, community forensic psychiatric nurses (CFPNs) and social workers play a pivotal role in assessment and discharge planning as well as maintaining and supporting individuals, their families and carers through subsequent life experiences. Community staff may be involved in the initial assessment stages right through to the restoration of good mental health, relapse prevention and the provision of crisis intervention, when required, 24 hours a day.

The process of preparing to move back into the community commences shortly after initial admission to hospital or even before by careful planning for later gradual re-introduction to life outside again. It may be a lengthy process for those who have been in various institutions, such as prison, special hospital or other facilities prior to admission to medium security. It can be stressful, particularly if family ties have been severed and meaningful relationships damaged or broken. Rehabilitation aims to increase confidence by assisting in relearning old skills and acquiring new ones in order, where possible, to enable the individual to live independently. Where this is not practicable extra support, for instance in a hostel environment, may be required with individuals and hostel staff being supported by the community forensic nurse and social workers.

This rehabilitation includes identifying appropriate accommodation resources. It means ensuring individuals are living in a suitable circumstances and that they have daytime activities such as a day centre, drop-in clubs, or are undertaking education, training or employment. It also aims to maximise the individual's financial entitlement. It includes an assessment of risk, in which the individual's independence is involved but not at the expense of the protection of the general public.

In medium secure units CFPN departments consist frequently of nurses qualified in forensic and community nursing. Each may work within a specific clinical team and contribute to the overall provision of follow-up care to individuals prior to and following discharge into the community. The CFPN department is inextricably linked with the social work department as well as other multidisciplinary team members to provide a pro-active response to the care of mentally disordered offenders and also to participate in developments in the field of forensic mental health care generally.

The challenge of working with an individual with mental health problems in the community is in maintaining a relationship aiming to prevent relapse into mental illness and associated disorganised or dangerous behaviour. All factors are influenced by circumstances such as family and social situations, cultural and spiritual matters, institutional factors and life events. Empathic understanding of individuals and their circumstances with a non-judgemental approach is crucial to facilitate personal growth. Recognition of each patient as unique is the grounding on which to base programmes of care and support which improve lifestyle and coping strategies. The role of the CFPN and social work in relation to the needs of the mentally disordered offenders may be subject to many influences, including clinical issues, public interests and the relevant statutory law. The following may be seen as key elements in the development of this role:

- Provision of comprehensive psychiatric assessment along with other multidisciplinary team members.
- Provision of nursing and social work intervention.
- Taking the key worker role to coordinate care provision under the Care Programme Approach (CPA).
- Establishment of links with local services, families and relevant agencies.
- Ensuring legal requirements of any relevant legislation are met.
- Twenty-four-hour responsibility for a caseload.
- Participation in a 24-hour on-call service to individuals and their carers.
- Supporting diversion/liaison services in police stations, magistrates courts and prisons.
- Advising other agencies in the criminal justice system, such as the probation service and bail hostels.
- Provision of education and training to other professions.
- Research and other academic pursuits.

Multiprofessional working

For an effective and comprehensive assessment to take place, open multiprofessional working is essential for the benefit of this client group. The initial in-patient assessment and later meetings with referring agencies and others should allow for discussion of future placements. The community team members will further assess and interview the patient to obtain further details of family members, team members etc. and views about where the patient would eventually like to live.

Occupational therapy involvement, to determine an individual's level of social functioning, is a vital component when the clinical team are selecting appropriate accommodation options. The CFPN and social worker work closely together in the community. Each has their own specific responsibilities, but some 'blurring' of roles may occur.

The CFPN will aim to provide comprehensive nursing care within the community as part of a multiprofessional clinical team. Their main tasks include establishing rapport with the patient whilst in the secure setting, to develop links with the patient's carers and relevant agencies with which they are involved, to have key worker role responsibility and to implement the Care Programme Approach and risk assessment. CFPNs administer prescribed medication, monitor compliance, perform psychiatric nursing assessment and provide professional advice to others.

The specific role of the forensic social worker is outlined in *Forensic Social Worker Competence and Workforce* (Central Council for Education and Training in Social Work, 1995). In brief, the key purpose of a forensic social worker is to hold in balance the protection of the general public and the promotion of the quality of life of mentally disordered offenders. The main tasks of a forensic social worker are assessment, care planning and management, report writing, working with individuals and families, managing crisis and trauma, maintaining effective social supervision, managing external systems and undertaking complementary professional activities. These tasks are all undertaken from an anti-oppressive perspective.

Community forensic care philosophy

Forensic psychiatric patients in the community should ideally be supported by multiprofessional teams in which psychiatrists, nurses, social workers, psychologists, occupational therapists all play a role.

A CPA framework is adopted to ensure comprehensive assessment, regular review and to fulfil the identified roles of each member of the team, including that of the allocated key worker. Discharge plans are commenced at an early stage and include assessment of risk both to the individual and general public, with planned strategies for risk management. The period following admission and during the early assessment stage is an anxious time for family and carers, and community staff can use this period of time to provide the necessary support to them and assess the home situation. It may not always be possible for the individual to return to the family but support systems can be identified and families can be encouraged to participate in the planning of future care provision. It is also an opportunity to provide education about the effects of mental illness and hospitalisation, particularly if it is given to family members who may have been the victim of the offence but still feel loyal to their relative. It is crucial for community staff to be involved during the early stages of admission, not only to have a detailed knowledge of the individual but because a familiar face in a crisis after discharge can often diffuse tense situations. A main role of the forensic community worker is to persuade and reassure both families and accommodation providers, that when caring for forensic patients, support will always be available. The specialist nature of forensic mental health lends itself to a consistent approach. This philosophy is based on the notion of collective 24-hour care. Individual clinical teams may have relatively smaller caseloads than in general psychiatry. This enables community workers to develop therapeutic relationships with the patients and their carers. It also allows for patients to be supported according to need. If required, a 24-hour duty team can provide additional monitoring and support and if the situation warrants, community workers can coordinate and initiate respite care at times of crisis.

CFPN caseloads consist of offenders with a range of mental health problems and psychiatric diagnoses and number between fifteen and twenty patients. This is fewer than community mental health nurses in other fields due to the intensive degree of support required. The geographical spread of work is also wider. Approximately two-thirds of the caseload may consist of individuals who are informal and agreeable to continued follow-up and psychiatric treatment. The remainder may be subject to restriction orders. These are individuals who have committed imprisonable offences who have been given a Hospital Order but because there has been concern for the protection of public safety, restrictions have also been placed on discharge. This places the ultimate authority for transfer or discharge of a patient with the government minister. It also has implications for the individual after discharge from hospital. There may be conditions, such as where they can live, what type of work they can do alongside other aspects of their treatment and aftercare.

Accommodation for mentally disordered offenders

During the rehabilitation of the mentally disordered offender careful consideration and strategies are adopted to gain the support of accommodation providers. Patients discharged from a secure setting may cause heightened anxiety in the community where they are to live. It is potentially difficult to find accommodation resources for some people who have committed serious crimes and who have the stigma of both offending and serious mental health problems.

The first task of community workers is to identify the range of resources available. Visits are made to accommodation establishments and preliminary discussions are undertaken to explore the feasibility of potential placements. Where patients eventually live can depend heavily on local knowledge. Some resources or directories of resources may be available through local authority social services departments, voluntary agencies or the private sector. With appropriate regard for confidentiality and consent where necessary, potential accommodation providers are furnished with reports from all disciplines regarding the individual's history, the index offence and risk assessment. This helps to maintain an open and honest relationship with patients and potential support staff. Multiprofessional case conferences are convened to discuss the proposed placements. The accommodation providers will meet the client and this enables them to complete their own assessment. The patient will have an opportunity to view the accommodation on offer. This may include a number of visits to enable a therapeutic relationship to be established as well as offering a comprehensive period of assessment.

The period of identifying and securing accommodation can be extremely time-consuming. Even when the placement has been agreed a further assessment period of four to eight weeks may be necessary before a placement can be considered permanent. Owing to the stigma of mental health and the nature of their offences, i.e. murder, arson, manslaughter and assault etc., it may prove undesirable or impossible to rehabilitate some mentally disordered offenders back into the community from which they came. This may be due to a variety of reasons, including protection of victims or restrictions imposed by the Home Office. Some patients, for instance those who have been in medium security or special hospitals for some considerable time, may become institutionalised. They, like others, may require long-term 24-hour psychiatric intervention in specialised mental health resources not provided by local services. This may include residential care homes, rehabilitation hostels, or private sector accommodation.

Discharge planning

At the stage of discharge planning the clinical team, along with other interested parties, meet to discuss statutory aftercare and community supervision. They will review the ongoing risk assessment and fine tune the community care plan, which will include the roles and responsibilities of each clinical team member. In addition, the clinical team will outline their expectations of the patient in relation to their follow-up in the community. This plan may be reviewed as necessary and at three-monthly CPA case conferences.

The aftercare plan must be reviewed regularly, which includes the assessment of risk. The aims of this are to identify whether the patient is a significant risk of seriously harming themselves or others as a result of enduring mental illness, if there are signs indicative of relapse, and what action to take in the event of any change in circumstances when discharged into the community under the care of the responsible medical officer and supervision of the social supervisor (social worker), provided that they adhere to specified conditions.

Community follow-up

The frequency of contact by the community workers is clearly outlined within CPA documentation. However, small caseloads allow community workers to increase levels of direct involvement, and intervention, as required. This facilitates frequent monitoring of the patient's mental health as well as giving of advice and support regarding social, financial and other matters. Community workers also spend a considerable amount of their professional time liaising with other agencies, carers and other clinical team members, in order to ensure that the individual patient's case and care plan is always under review. This allows them to highlight problems as early as possible and prevent a further relapse in mental health or offending behaviour. Through the interactions between the community workers and patients, assessment and monitoring take place.

The overall objectives of the community worker are to enable the patient to achieve their ultimate level of functioning within the community. The clinical team attempts to assist the patient to progress through the rehabilitation process from hospital to hostel or semi-independent living if and when appropriate, and then to independent accommodation and living.

Clearly not every patient is able to achieve this end. They may periodically relapse and move back some way temporarily. The rehabilitation process is a long-term activity requiring a flexible approach from the community forensic services in response to the changing needs of the individual.

When patients remain mentally stable but continue to be involved in criminal activity they may remain in the criminal justice system and be monitored there by members of the community services linked to local prisons. Some may continue to be in contact with forensic services for many years. Others may pass to the care of other teams. In some cases it may be appropriate to collaborate with psychiatric services to provide a model of joint care, either over a transitional period or in the longer term.

Case study

A 21-year-old male was admitted to hospital as an involuntary patient after a psychotic episode when he became paranoid about a close friend, believing that he was going to be killed. He had attacked his friend with a knife and was subsequently charged with wounding. During the time he spent in hospital all his friends remained loyal to him, realising that the assault was due to mental illness. It was evident that there had been concern about him for some time prior to the offence. With treatment his symptoms resolved and his friends became involved in the arrangements for his aftercare. They were given information also to contact members of the clinical team . With the support of his friends, his family were also able to be involved despite living a considerable distance away.

Some, but not all, aspects of assertive outreach are adopted in the overall model of provision in the community with a team approach. Persistence in maintaining contact with individuals, particularly if there are early warning signs of relapse or when there is a reluctance to engage or continue with follow-up, is necessary. A team approach is also more effective at providing appropriate care in the community. It can provide support for individual workers who may be inclined to readmission when difficulties arise, without a supportive team around them. Teams can also provide more effective clinical supervision as each team member has a familiarity with individuals on the caseload and will be aware of relevant issues.

Case study

A 31-year-old woman had a long history of in-patient care following transfer from a female prison to a special hospital and then to a medium secure unit for rehabilitation to prepare for living more independently in the community. She had a diagnosis of personality disorder and a history of self-harm, ranging from minor injury to life-threatening situations. Due to the seriousness of her index offence she was subject to a restriction order and discharge plans had to be approved by the Home Office. She moved into a hostel with a comprehensive care plan which was devised to involve input from most members of the multidisciplinary team, as well as other agencies. This detailed her care and treatment as well as plans for education, social and recreational needs. Initially she had difficulty settling outside an institutional setting and for some time was frequently in crisis, requiring the involvement of on-call services. She was ambivalent about follow-up care and reluctant to accept visits from staff who were working with her. On occasions she acted upon her threats of self-harm in order to reduce her level of stress. With daily visits from community staff and with the support of the whole team having input into her care, she was eventually able to gain in confidence and progress towards a more independent life. Whilst she had frequent re-admissions to hospital in the initial stages, these reduced in number over time and with the support she received.

Summary

Discharge from hospital is a significant event for both the patient and carer. To ensure good practice, discharge should not be a matter of chance. Rehabilitation from secure conditions starts from the moment a referral and planned admission has been agreed. The process is on-going and continually evolving according to the needs of the patient, their family and the wider community, as well as the availability of suitable accommodation and local resources. The multiprofessional team will attempt to work to an agreed plan in arranging care and necessary support for eventual discharge. In accordance with the Care Programme Approach each team member's role and responsibility in the rehabilitation of the patient will be identified. The team should work in a cohesive manner to ensure effective communication, thus aiming to minimise the risk of a breakdown in care following discharge. Due to the risk factors associated with the care of this client group a complex and resource-intensive discharge care package will be required. It is important that the best use of health and social care resources is made, as the consequences of errors and poor practice may be great to the patient, carers, community and service provider.

References

Blackburn, R. (1992) Criminal behaviour, personality disorder and mental illness. The origins of confusion. *Criminal Behaviour and Mental Health*, 2, pp. 66–77.

Blom-Cooper, L., Hally, H. and Murphy, E. (1995) *The Falling Shadow: One Patients Mental Health Care*. Duckworth, London.

Blom-Cooper, L., Grounds, A. and Guinan, P. (1966) The Case of Jason Mitchell. Report of the Independent Panel of Inquiry. Duckworth, London.

Central Council for Education and Training in Social Work (1995) *Forensic Social Worker Competence and Workforce* CCETSW: London.

Coid, J. (1991) 'Difficult to place' psychiatric patients. *British Medical Journal*, 302, pp. 603–4.

Collins, A., Hill, O. and Taylor, M. (1994) Independent Inquiry into Kevin Rooney. North East Thames Regional Health Authority.

Crichton, J. (ed.) (1995b) *Psychiatric Patient Violence: Risk and Response*. Duckworth, London.

Crichton, J. (1995a) *The Falling Shadow*: Comments on the Robinson Inquiry. *Psychiatric Care*, 2 (5) 175–9.

Department of Health (1990) The Care Programme Approach. Department of Health Circular HC (90) 23 LASSL (90). 11 September 1990.

Department of Health (1996) Confidential Inquiry into Homicides and Suicides by Mentally Ill People (The Boyd Report). HMSO, London.

Department of Health and the Home Office (1992) Review of Health and Social Services for Mentally Disordered Offenders and Others Requiring Similar Services (Chairman: Dr John Reed). HMSO, London.

Dick, D., Shuttleworth, B. and Charlton, J. (1990) Report of the Panel of Inquiry Appointed by West Midlands Regional Health Authority and the Special Hospital Service Authority to Investigate the Case of Kim Kirkman. West Midlands Regional Health Authority.

Heginbotham, C., Hale, R., Warren, L., Walsh, T. and Carr, J. (1994) Report of the Independent Panel of Inquiry Examining the Case of Michael Buchanan. North West London Mental Health NHS Trust.

Home Office (1990) Provision for Mentally Disordered Offenders. Circular 66/90.

Home Office (1992) House of Commons Health Committee: Community Supervision Orders. Health Committee 5th Report, Vol. 1. HMSO, London.

Home Office (1993) Community Care Reforms and the Criminal Justice System. Circular 29/93.

Home Office (1995) Mental Health (Patients in the Community) Act. Guidance on Supervised Discharge (Aftercare Under Supervision) and Related Provisions. HMSO, London.

Home Office and Department of Health (1994) Report by the Working Group on Psychopathic Disorder (Reed *et al.*). HMSO, London.

Repper, J. and Perkins, R. (1995) Targeting services for seriously mentally ill people: implications for Community Psychiatric Nurses. In C. Brooker and E. White (eds), *Community Psychiatric Nursing: A Research Prospective*, Vol. 3. Chapman & Hall, London.

Ritchie, J.H. (Chairman), Dick, D. and Lingham, R. (1994) The Report of the Inquiry into the Care and Treatment of Christopher Clunis. HMSO, London.

Spokes, J., Pare, M. and Royle, G. (1988) Report of the Committee of Inquiry into the Care and Aftercare of Sharon Campbell. HMSO, London.

Future challenges

Norman McClelland, Martin Humphreys and Lorraine Conlon

Forensic mental health care is still a relatively young and developing area. Much of what has changed over the years, at least in the United Kingdom, has come about as a result of reaction to adverse events and, in some cases, disaster. Clinical practice has had, necessarily, to progress rapidly, but frequently in difficult, restrictive and, at times, hostile environments. Caring for difficult, disruptive, rejected and sometimes dangerous individuals may take its toll, and can also result in stigmatisation for health care workers, as well as patients, even within their own professional groups. There is, nevertheless, still much to be done in the field. There are huge challenges now facing forensic services from a practical, clinical and political point of view. There have been calls for major changes in service provision for mentally disordered people, not least those who fall foul of the criminal justice system, and are perceived as a danger to society.

In terms of specific issues, the clearly identified need for longer term, medium secure, facilities is something which now needs to be addressed as a matter of urgency. Currently the majority of this form of care is available only through the independent sector, although there are various initiatives under way around the country, particularly in England and Wales, to provide for those who require more than the two years in medium security, which current regional services aim to work to. This group, most frequently those suffering from chronic, intractable and treatment-resistant psychotic illness, in some ways typify the subsets of patients who gravitate towards secure psychiatric hospitals, for whatever reason, but for whom there have been relatively few specific and tailored forms of care and therapy. Others who pose a real challenge to services and service providers include female patients, who are very much in the minority in secure psychiatric hospitals, those from ethnic minority groups, particularly those which are over-represented when compared to the general population, such as black African Caribbean males, patients with a primary diagnosis of learning disability, but who also need secure care, and lastly those with severe personality disorder. Each of these groups of patients have particular needs, which, even with the best will in the world, still need to be identified by careful research and investigation, and then addressed. Another area which is important in this context is the increasing recognition of the need for so-called user involvement in consultation over the whole range of issues in patient care and research into mental disorder as a whole, and particularly the care of detained patients and those who require secure confinement.

Mental health legislation is set to change throughout the United Kingdom. Major review of existing law is under way at the beginning of the new millennium, and this will inevitably lead to differences. There is no doubt that this will affect the care and treatment of certain mentally disordered offenders and others who require similar services, although somewhat paradoxically, this may be less so than for patients made subject to compulsory measures through criminal rather than civil procedures. In the current political climate it does seem that detention in hospital, and compulsory treatment in the community, may become more restrictive for those involuntary patients who have not come through the criminal justice system, and thus come to reflect more closely those committed to hospital by the courts.

The term 'dangerous severe personality disorder' has gained political recognition in the wake of some high profile cases. The Committee of Inquiry into the personality disorder unit at Ashworth Hospital (Fallon *et al.*, 1999) did find some consistency and value in the term 'severe personality disorder' for clinical purposes. It is unclear as yet whether these two terms might mean the same thing, or refer to the same clinical entity, but deliberations over the former are likely to have a major impact for the group of individuals so identified, and it does seem likely that psychiatric and allied services will inevitably be required to be involved.

Perhaps most importantly of all, there is a continuing need, particularly for public, but also professional education in relation to the needs of mentally disordered people who need care in a secure environment. Without a constant awareness and recognition of the stigma associated with both psychiatric disorder and offending behaviour, and an overriding commitment to break it down, the future of secure care will be limited, and the lives of those passing through will remain little altered or improved.

Reference

Fallon, P., Bluglass, R., Edwards, B. and Daniels, G. (1999) The Report of the Committee of Inquiry into the Personality Disorder Unit, Ashworth Special Hospital. Cm 4194-11. The Stationery Office, London.

Index

Accommodation:
  probation hostel, 121–3
  during rehabilitation, 133–4
Activities, 58
Admission:
  declining, 7–8
  staffing levels, 9
Aftercare, 127–37
  accommodation, 133–4
  follow-up, 134–5
  team working, 28–31, 131–2
  see also Community care, 132
Aggression, 42–72
  in context, 44–5
  de-escalation, 16, 59–67
  defined, 44
  post-incident debriefing, 67–8
  post-incident review, 69
  prevention, 45–59
  recording and reporting, 68–9
  theories, 44
All Saints Hospital, Birmingham, 35
Anger management, 16
Assessment, 1, 11–20, 49, 52
  case study, 17, 18
  dimensions, 12, 13
  groups, 13
  of risk, 14–19
  tools, 17, 19
Audit, 68
Autonomy, 63

Bail hostel, 121–3
Bail information officer, 119
Beck Depression Inventory, 36
Behaviour identification, 55
Behavioural Status Index, 19
Beneficence, 45
Blackwood, O., 17
Buchanan, M., 128
Building design, 8, 58

Campbell, S., 128

Care in the community, 99–102, 127, 132–3,
  134–5
Care Programme Approach, 100, 128
Carers, 21–8
  support groups, 24–7
Case studies:
  assessment, 17, 18
  community care, 135
  de-escalation, 66
  referral, 7, 8
  self-harm, 81, 88
  violence continuum, 52
Childhood experiences, 85–6
Client-centred care, 16, 35–6
Clinical supervision, 107–8
Clunis, C., 17, 100, 127
Collaboration, 30, 31
Colour, 58
Communication, 57, 60–3
  non-verbal, 61–3
  in team working, 30–1
  verbal, 61
Community care, 99–102, 127, 132–3, 134–5
Community Forensic Psychiatric Nurse
  (CFPN), 117, 122, 130–1, 132–3
Community Psychiatric Nurse (CPN), 114,
  115
Community Treatment (Supervision)
  Orders, 102, 103
Compliance, 6, 53
Conditional discharge, 130
Consent, 99
Contraband, 55
Control and restraint 46–8, see also Physical
  restraint
Counselling, 65
Court diversion, 116–19
Court probation officer, 118–19
Criminal history, 4, 15
Crown Prosecutor, 118
Custody, diversion from, 113–16

Dangerous severe personality disorder, 139

De-briefing, 67–8
De-escalation, 16, 59–67
Detention, 97–9
Developmental history, 2, 4
Diaries, 17
Discharge:
  conditional, 130
  planning, 134
  supervised, 129
Diversion, 113–26
  from court 116–19
  economic factors, 123–4
  effectiveness, 124
  at point of arrest, 113–16
  from prison, 119–20
  support workers, 120
Diversionary activities, 65
Duty of care, 43

'Early Signs', 35
Education and training, 46–9, 56, 105–12
  control and restraint, 46–8
  post-registration, 108–9
  training trainers, 48–9
  university sector, 109–12
Elliot House, 121–3
English National Board, 108
Environmental factors, 8–9, 11, 58–9
Ethics, 45
Ethnicity and self-harm, 87
Eye contact, 62–3

'Falling Shadow, The', 127, 128
Family, 15, 21–8
  support groups, 24–7
Forensic medical examiner, 115

Gender and self-harm, 83–4
Genuineness, 56
Group:
  assessment, 13
  psychoeducational, 34–8
  Self-Injury Group, 80–1
  support for relatives, 24–7
  therapy, 16, 37–8

Health and Safety at Work Act (1974), 45
Health policy, 99–102
History, 2, 4
Holding powers, 97–9
Honesty, 56
Hostels, 121–3
Hybrid Order, 129

Incident forms, 68–9
Index offence, 15
Induction programmes, 106–7
Inquiries and reports, 17, 100, 119, 127–31
Insight Assessment Scale, 36, 38
Intervention plans, 15–16
Interviews, 5–7

Joint Board of Clinical Nursing Studies, 108
Judgemental attitudes, 57

Legal aspects, 97–104
Listening, 61

Management of Health and Safety at Work
  Regulations, 45
Medication cards, 6
Mental Health (Patients in the Community)
  Act (1995), 101
Mitchell, J., 128
Motivation, 56
Multiprofessional teams, *see* Team working

Needs assessment, 52, 54
Negotiation, 63
Noise, 58
Non-maleficence, 45
Non-verbal communication, 61–3
Normalisation, 127

Observation, 53–5, 90
Occupation, 31–2
Occupational therapy, 58, 131
Offending behaviour, 4, 15
Outside contact, 59

Pace of life, 59
Patients:
  care involvement, 53
  environmental needs, 58–9
  information for, 53, 55
  outside contact, 59
  privacy, 59
  relationships with professionals, 40–1
Personal space, 62
Personality disorders, 139
Physical restraint 46–8, 67, 70
  monitoring forms, 69
Placement, appropriateness, 52–3
Police and Criminal Evidence Act (1984),
  114
Police custody, diversion from, 113–16
Post-registration training, 108–9
Power of detention, 97–9
Preceptorship, 107
Pre-vocational programmes, 34
Prison:
  diversion, 119–20
  mental health screening, 120
  reception, 120
Privacy, 59
Probation hostel, 121–3
Probation officers, 118–19
Probation service, 129
Problem solving, 65
Professional–patient relationships, 40–1
Professionalism, 56
Project 2000, 109
Prosecution, 118

Psychiatric history, 4
Psychoeducation, 34–9
'PUNCH', 49, 50

Reaside Clinic, 80, 106, 108, 109
Reed Report, 119, 128
Referral:
  case studies, 7, 8
  letters, 5
  source, 1
  urgent, 2
Rehabilitation, 130, 133
  vocational, 31–4
Relatives, 15, 21–8
  support groups, 24–7
Reports and inquiries, 17, 100, 119, 127–31
Resources, 58
Restriction order, 129–30
Risk assessment 14–19
Risk Assessment, Management and Audit
  System, 19
Ritchie Report, 17, 100, 127–8
Robinson, A., 128
Rooney, K., 128

Safety, 6–7, 8, 42, 43, 45, 58
  risk assessment, 14–19
  see also Aggression
Schizophrenia, psychoeducation model, 34–9
Security levels, 55, *see also* Safety
Self-harm, 73–96
  activities, 88–9
  case studies, 81, 88
  childhood experiences, 85–6
  contagious nature, 89
  defined, 74–7
  diagnosis and, 81–3
  ethnicity, 87
  function, 87–8
  gender, 83–4
  management, 89–93
  medication, 91
  negative attitudes towards, 78–81
  onset, 84–6
  prevalence, 77–8
  terminology, 74–5
  time-of-day, 88

Self-Injury Group, 80–1
Self-mutilation, 75
Self-report, 17
Severe personality disorder, 139
Sexual abuse, 85–6
Social workers, 130–1, 132
Staff induction, 106–7
Statutory duties, 97–9
STEP initiative, 34
Suicide, *see* Self-harm
Supervised discharge, 129
Supervision, clinical, 107–8
Supervision registers, 128

Team working, 2, 6, 9, 28–31
  advantages, 29
  aftercare, 131–2
  collaboration, 30, 31
  communication, 30–1
  consistency, 57
  daily discussions, 68
  defined, 28–9
  drawbacks, 29–30
  leadership, 29
  self-harm management, 91–2
Terminal illness, 40
Therapeutic alliance, 53
Training, *see* Education and training
Treatment, 21–41
  aggression considerations, 63–5
  compliance, 6, 53
  consent to, 99
  dilemmas, 39–41
  groups, 16, 37–8

University education, 109–12

Verbal communication, 61
Victoria Law Courts, Birmingham, 117–18
Violence, 42–3, 44
  continuum, 49, 51, 52, 59
  see also Aggression
Vocational rehabilitation, 31–4

Winson Green Prison, 119–20
Work, 31–2
Workplace Regulations, 45